MW01200531

Diabetes Type 2
You can reverse it naturally
Lose weight and restore your health

Sandra Cabot MD

Margaret Jasinska ND

Diabetes Type 2 - You can reverse it naturally. Lose weight and restore your health

Copyright © 2007 Dr Sandra Cabot and Margaret Jasinska ND

Revised and printed in the United States of America in 2011

Published by
SCB International Inc.
PO Box 5070 Glendale AZ USA 85312
Phone 623 334 3232

www.liverdoctor.com
www.weightcontroldoctor.com

ISBN: 978-0-982-93362-6

1) Diabetes 2) Nutrition 3) Diet 4) Health

Contents

Introduction 5

1. Basic information about Diabetes 14

    What is Diabetes? 14

    Functions of insulin 15

    Types of Diabetes 18

2. Risk factors and symptoms of
Diabetes 21

    Risk factors for developing Type 2 Diabetes 21

    Symptoms of Diabetes 31

    Skin signs of Syndrome X and
    Type 2 Diabetes 32

3. Tests to diagnose and monitor
Diabetes 34

    Who should be tested for Diabetes? 34

    Blood tests to diagnose Type 2 Diabetes 35

    Essential ongoing tests to monitor Diabetes 38

    Checking your blood sugar level yourself
    at home 43

    Summary of essential tests for diabetics 44

4. The health complications of Diabetes 47

    The main complications of Diabetes are: 47

5. Medication used in the treatment of Type 2 Diabetes ...58

6. Reversing Type 2 Diabetes through diet 62

    All about protein 62

    All about Fat 66

    All about Carbohydrate 72

    What about glycemic index (GI)? 73

    Artificial sweeteners 76

    Specific beneficial foods for diabetics 79

7. Conventional dietary recommendations for diabetics
and why they'll make you worse 82

    The diet advice you've been given and
    why it's making you worse 82

8. Reversing Type 2 Diabetes through
   lifestyle changes 86
   The importance of exercise 86
   Sleep 88
   Stress management 90
   Coping with depression 92
9. Reversing Type 2 Diabetes through
   nutritional and herbal medicine 94
   Helpful Supplements for Diabetics 94
   Antioxidants 99
10. Specific recommendations for
    avoiding diabetic complications 102
11. Eating plan to reverse type 2
    Diabetes 106
    Foods you can eat 106
    Beverages 112
    Foods that must be avoided
    on the eating plan 115
    Portion Sizes 116
    Avoiding Hypoglycemia (low blood sugar) 119
    Diabetic 2 week meal plan 121
12. Recipes to reverse Type 2 Diabetes 124
    Breakfast recipes 124
    Lunch recipes 132
    Dinner recipes 140
    Vegetarian Recipes 148
    Maintenance: how to keep Diabetes at bay 154
    Type 1 Diabetes in more detail 155
    Diet guidelines for Type 1 Diabetics 157
Conclusion 159
Glossary 160
References 163
Index 166

Introduction

Diabetes is a serious disease; it can shorten your life and create many chronic health problems unless well managed. Diabetes is also an epidemic; it now affects approximately 246 million people worldwide, with 46 percent of them in the 40 to 59 years age group. The prediction is that the number of people living with Diabetes will skyrocket to 380 million in the next 20 years if current trends continue.

There are two main types of Diabetes: type 1 Diabetes, which generally develops in childhood and requires the use of insulin injections, and Type 2 Diabetes, which typically affects middle aged overweight adults and is controlled by diet or tablets. The incidence of both types of Diabetes is rising, but it is Type 2 Diabetes that is really escalating out of control. Approximately 8.3 percent of the population of the USA has Diabetes. Type 2 Diabetes accounts for 85 to 90 percent of all cases of Diabetes.

Type 2 Diabetes is referred to as a lifestyle disease, because it is largely a result of poor diet, obesity and an inactive lifestyle. It is well known that we are in the middle of an obesity epidemic, and the rise in Type 2 Diabetes is just a natural consequence of this. Many people don't realize what a serious disease Diabetes is; it can lead to blindness, kidney failure, amputations, erectile dysfunction, heart attacks and strokes. Four out of five people with Diabetes die of heart disease. The longer you are a diabetic, the more likely you are to develop complications of the disease. Therefore, the younger you are when diagnosed the worse off you will be.

The most frightening thing about Type 2 Diabetes is its recent emergence in children. The disease used to be called adult onset Diabetes because it was unheard of in children; this is not the case anymore; in the last ten years it has become the biggest threat to the health of American children. Children as young as eight years old are being diagnosed with the disease. Because children are developing a disease of middle age, this is the first generation where children may die before their parents.

The ironic thing is that Type 2 Diabetes is a preventable disease; you don't have to become a diabetic! Even if you have a strong family history of it, you can prevent yourself from becoming a diabetic. If you have already been diagnosed with Type 2 Diabetes, lifestyle changes and nutritional medicine can reverse the disease in the majority of cases. You can eliminate your requirement for medication and normalize your blood sugar, or at the very least reduce your requirement for medication, if you make the necessary changes to your life. As long as your pancreas can still produce insulin, our eating plan can reverse most cases of Type 2 Diabetes.

This book focuses mostly on Type 2 Diabetes, so unless we state differently, we are generally referring to Type 2 Diabetes throughout the book. We disagree with much of the dietary advice given to diabetics and believe it actually contributes to making the disease worse. A typical scenario is where a person is diagnosed with Type 2 Diabetes; their doctor tells them they must lose weight and refers them to a Diabetes educator. The patient is given specific dietary advice to follow and sent home.

It is almost impossible to lose weight if you are a diabetic and follow the recommended high carbohydrate, low fat diet. A diet like this will make it hard to keep your blood sugar down and, in fact, over the years your blood sugar will rise and you will probably have to go on tablets to control it. Over time, the dose of your medication will be raised, and a few unfortunate individuals with Type 2 Diabetes may have to go on insulin therapy. All the while you will continue to gain weight. These are all clear signs that a disease is getting worse; if you follow the recommended low fat, high carbohydrate diet there is every chance that your Diabetes will get worse. The eating plan in this book will help to lower your blood sugar and insulin levels, plus will help you to lose weight.

Diabetes presents a huge economic burden on individuals, the community and the government. The United States government spends more money on Diabetes than any other health condition. In 2007, Diabetes cost the country approximately $174 billion; the cost is sure to have risen since then. It is predicted the Diabetes epidemic will greatly hinder the economic growth of many developed and developing nations.

In this book we give you the knowledge and tools to prevent or reverse Type 2 Diabetes. If you are a diabetic, the better informed you are about your health, the less likely you are to succumb to the long term complications of the disease.

I think this book will be a great help to the millions of people who now suffer with Diabetes type two for several reasons –

• It will give them understanding and knowledge and remove confusion.

• It will give them practical tools to prevent and even reverse this awful disease.

• It will awaken their bodies and minds to a new way of eating.

• It will provide them with an overall strategy to not only live longer but to achieve a real sense of mental and physical wellbeing.

The knowledge in this book is based on many years of clinical experience and research and we have great confidence in our program. You, as a reader and consumer of this program can only achieve the confidence we have after you have tried the way of eating and lifestyle changes in this book. Then you will see for yourself the amazing benefits and changes in your metabolism, which will show up as –

• Sustained weight loss

• Sustained reductions in your blood sugar and insulin levels

• Increased energy levels

Our philosophy and methods may challenge the advice that you have been given by conventional dieticians and other weight loss books. If you have tried these more conventional approaches to little or no avail, we are not surprised, as we have found that they do not work for the majority of overweight and/or diabetic patients. This is why we have written this book which we believe will hold the key to success for people who are sick and tired of being sick and tired.

Over the years we have found that many of our patients find it difficult to understand the physiology behind the control of the metabolism of fat and sugar in the body. This lack of understanding creates an obstacle to successful and easy control of weight and blood sugar levels. I will now attempt to describe the way the body controls the levels of fat and sugar in the body by using a simple analogy.

The hormone known as insulin controls the use of fats and sugars by the cells in your body. The pancreas gland produces insulin and secretes it into the bloodstream. Fats and sugars get absorbed from the intestines into the bloodstream after eating a meal. The fats and the sugars are converted into physical energy inside the cells and this energy enables the cells to perform their functions. The question must be asked – how do the fats and sugars get inside the cells where they can be used for energy? The answer is – insulin transports them into the inside of the cells.

I like to describe insulin as a motor car and the fat and the sugar as the passengers inside the motor car. The fats and sugars cannot enter the cells by themselves – they need to be transported into the cells by a motor car called insulin. The motor car must enter the cell via a special gate in the cell membrane which opens to let the passengers disembark inside the cell. This gateway is the receptor for insulin and is situated on the cell membrane.

If the gateway or the motor car do not work properly, the fats and sugars cannot enter inside the cells and they accumulate in the bloodstream. Thus the blood sugar rises too much and the pancreas responds by making more and more insulin and the result is too much insulin. However, the insulin does not work properly and the gateway into the cell will not open. Thus the blood sugar continues to rise and the cells are starved of the sugar they need for energy production.

If the sugar cannot get inside the cell, the motor car will take it somewhere else – in this case the insulin motor car takes the sugar to the liver or fat tissues and turns it into fat. Yes that's right – sugar gets turned into fat instead of energy. The results are –

- You put on weight
- You get a fatty liver
- You feel tired and crave more sugar

Now you see how insulin is a fat storing hormone and if you produce too much insulin you will store more fat.

Most people get fat on a diet that is not high in fat and they don't understand why. It's not the number of calories that matters so much, it is the source of the calories.

We must get the motor car and the gateway working efficiently to lower blood sugar and convert dietary fat and sugar into energy.

Welcome to the new world of an efficient metabolism where sugar is more efficiently used for energy and not for the storage of body fat.

Testimonial

I interviewed Barry about his long struggle to control his weight and Diabetes and it really impressed me, as I could see the difficulty and frustrations he had overcome to be very successful. I thought to myself, not everybody could do this, you need to be committed and passionate about your health and you need discipline. Yes it's a huge challenge but Barry has done it. Barry is a surveyor and is a man who likes to understand the science and rationale behind the things he tries. Barry is now 57 years of age and is a healthy fit man who enjoys his life but for most of his life he was very overweight and suffered with Syndrome X.

As a teenager Barry was overweight and continued to gain more weight into adulthood. He played sports and tried to be healthy but he was always hungry and craved sugar. Barry drank several liters of soda pops everyday however he was always thirsty, which is a common symptom of Diabetes. He became angry easily and suffered with a bad temper, which was probably caused by wild fluctuations in his blood sugar. At the age of 30 he was diagnosed with very high blood pressure and started on anti-hypertensive drugs which brought his blood pressure down. He tried different types of meal replacement shakes but he was always hungry and craved sweets.

At the age of 50 Barry weighed 275 pounds (125 kilograms) and for his height of five foot seven (1.7 metres) this was way too much and put him into the obese range. He tried to fight his weight problem by exercising more and although he did not need to do the hard physical work that the younger surveyors did, he took every opportunity to bang in the pegs and other physical chores at work. He tried many types of diets and although he could get down to 90 kilograms, it did not last long and his weight gain would resume as he had an enormous hunger.

Barry loved cars and at the age of 50 he thought that like a motor car of a certain mileage he should have a physical overhaul. He told the doctor *"I am not a pig and I don't eat as much as my colleagues at work, so why am I overweight and tired?"*

The doctor put Barry on a diet of 1200 calories a day and after 3 months of sticking to this, he had only lost a meagre 2.2 pounds (one kilogram). Not surprising, as although the diet was low in calories, it consisted predominantly of carbohydrates such as bread, pasta and cereals and was low in fat.

The doctor was not impressed with Barry's weight loss and said to Barry "You are meant to write everything you eat in the food diary I have given you !" He offered Barry drugs to reduce the absorption of fat from his meals but warned him that he would get diarrhea and have to wear diapers.

Barry snapped – he said *"No way – I demand to see a specialist!"*

He had to wait quite a few months but finally got to see a heart specialist who gave him a clean bill of health. Although this was a great relief, Barry still did not have the answers to his ballooning weight and by the age of 54 he weighed 297 pounds (135 kilograms) and then he became too big for his scales to accurately measure his weight.

He then demanded to see another specialist and after a long wait he finally got to see an endocrinologist. The endocrinologist found that Barry had dark brown pigment under his arms and that this was a sign of Diabetes. Blood tests revealed elevated levels of blood sugar (glucose was 234mg/dL) and elevated levels of insulin (fasting insulin was 330). The endocrinologist told Barry he had Syndrome X which had caused Diabetes type 2 and he was told to register himself as a diabetic.

Barry was worried by this and did not register himself as a diabetic because he was a fighter and now he knew the problem, he was going to overcome it and reverse his Diabetes. He was put on a low glycemic diet and thought that this time he was going to beat his weight problem. Unfortunately after 3 months on the low glycemic diet, he was no better off. Unbelievable he thought – *"something is wrong and it's time to do my own research"*. Well done Barry !

Barry started to test different foods by measuring their effect on his blood sugar. He found that carbohydrates such as sugar, grains, cereals, flour, many fruits and even some vegetables such as carrots and peas spiked his blood sugar levels. It did not matter if the grains were processed, refined, wholegrain or whatever; they still caused his blood sugar levels to spike. Conversely protein foods like meat, eggs, cheese, seafood, nuts, as well as green vegetables had no effect on his blood sugar levels and they remained low.

Barry felt vindicated – yes, he knew he was not a cheat and he was not going crazy and that the conventional advice of the medical profession did not work for him. He could have taken drugs to lower his blood sugar levels but he knew that this would not control his weight problem.

So Barry's research continued and he read about the hormone insulin and how it controlled blood sugar levels and how it made him hungry if it was too high. He wanted to understand this chemical imbalance called Syndrome X and during his investigations he came across the book titled *Can't Lose Weight ? You could have Syndrome X*. Barry read the book and thought "yes, yes, yes, I am reading my life's story!"

Barry started on the eating plan in this book and followed Stage One, which is very low in carbohydrate and eliminates grains. Indeed, he was very strict with himself and ate no grains or sugar and found that his hunger went away. After 54 years of struggling he was no longer continually hungry. He ate lots of protein and vegetables and one piece of fruit daily. The weight started to come off him easily, even though he was eating plenty of food, but it was a different way of eating for a man who had been addicted to carbohydrates. In this book we have tailor-made the eating plan and nutritional recommendations specifically to diabetics. The eating plan is similar to that in the Syndrome X book but is targeted even more so to diabetics.

In July 2006, Barry suffered with an attack of gout and had to commence Zyloprim tablets to lower his uric acid levels. This worked for him and the gout is no longer a problem. Patients with Syndrome X are at a higher risk of gout and if they change to a high protein diet they may precipitate an attack. To offset this it is important to drink a lot of water and eat vegetables that alkalize the body – such as cucumber, celery, lettuce and bell pepper.

Barry continues to control his blood sugar levels and today his average readings for blood glucose are only 72 mg/dL (4 mmol/L). His insulin remains elevated at a level of 120, however it still controls his blood sugar levels very well. Thus Barry is no longer diabetic and today feels happy and fit at a normal weight of 194 pounds (88 kilograms).

His diet consists of mainly protein in the form of meat, cheese, plain yogurt, seafood, nuts, eggs, poultry and also green vegetables. He has one piece of fruit daily. Barry uses stevia as a natural sweetener and also the protein powder known as Synd-X Slimming protein powder. He is never hungry and his libido is good.

Occasionally when Barry visits friends or attends a special family event he allows himself a sweet treat or two, but this is not a regular thing. Barry has a family history of weight problems and Syndrome X and now he has discovered the key to weight control and good health he is sending his sister and his daughters to get the right type of help.

I have no doubt that Barry would have become an insulin dependant diabetic with diabetic complications in his older age. This is because his insulin levels remain too high. It has taken a lot of hard work and discipline for him to be successful and I admire him for this.

We may not all be as disciplined or strong as Barry but with the knowledge in this book you will find that your struggle with weight excess and/or Diabetes becomes much easier. This is because the power of nutritional medicine is amazing, it is life changing, it is life saving and even the drug companies are disconcerted by its rapid spread and popularity.

If you have any questions while reading this book or following our eating plan, please feel free to phone Dr Cabot's Health Advisory Service in Australia on 02 4655 8855 or in the USA on 623 334 3232 and speak to a naturopath. You will also find a great deal of up to date health information on our website: www.weightcontroldoctor.com

A Word of Caution

If you are a diabetic and intend on following the diet and nutritional advice in this book, please remember the following points:

• Tell your doctor about any diet changes you intend to make and keep in regular contact with your doctor.

• Do not try to self diagnose. If you suffer with some of the symptoms mentioned in this book, please discuss these with your doctor and have the appropriate tests to confirm the diagnosis.

• If you are taking prescription medication for Diabetes, using insulin or taking any other prescription drugs, do not discontinue their use or reduce your dose without speaking to your doctor first.

• Tell your doctor if you wish to start taking a nutritional or herbal supplement.

1. Basic information about Diabetes

What is Diabetes?

Diabetes is a disease that results in high blood sugar. Foods that contain carbohydrate are digested and broken down into sugar, or glucose, which is used by your body for energy. The pancreas is an organ that sits behind the lower part of your stomach and manufactures the hormone called insulin. Insulin helps to get glucose into your cells, where it is used for energy. People with Diabetes either do not produce enough insulin, or the insulin they make no longer works properly. This means excess glucose builds up in the bloodstream.

More about the pancreas

The pancreas is approximately 15 centimeters (six inches) long and weighs between 85 and 100 grams (3 to 3.5 ounces). It is often described as having three regions: the head, body and tail. The head of the pancreas is located very close to the first part of your small intestine (the duodenum). The body and tail of the pancreas extend towards the spleen.

The pancreas has two main functions:

• It manufactures and secretes digestive enzymes into the small intestine. These enzymes act to digest carbohydrate, protein and fat.

• It releases the hormones insulin and glucagon into the bloodstream. These two hormones have opposing effects in the body. Insulin is released in response to a rise in blood sugar and it allows the transfer of glucose from the bloodstream into the cells of the body. Glucose that cannot be used immediately for energy is stored as glycogen in muscle and liver cells for future use. The body only has a limited capacity to store glycogen; therefore excess glucose will then be converted into the type of fat called triglyceride, and stored as body fat. So we can say that insulin is released when you are well fed and it encourages the storage of fat. That is why insulin has been called a fat producing hormone.

Glucagon is released when blood glucose levels are low, such as in between meals. *It encourages the burning of body fat stores for energy.* Glucagon converts fat and protein into glucose and raises low blood sugar levels.

Diagram of the pancreas in relation to other abdominal organs

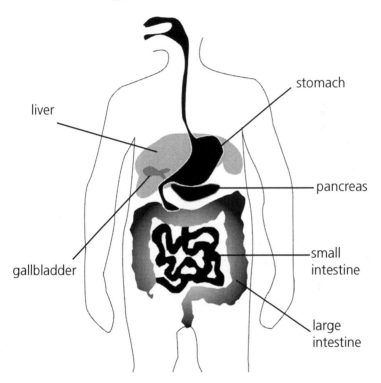

Functions of insulin

When you eat food containing carbohydrates (or sugars), this causes a rise in your blood sugar level. Your pancreas secretes insulin into your bloodstream in response to this rise in blood sugar (glucose). Most cells of the body have insulin receptors on their surface which bind with the insulin in circulation. These receptors are found on the cell membrane; that is why having healthy cell membranes is so important if you want to reverse Diabetes. When a cell has insulin attached to a receptor on its surface, the cell is able to absorb glucose from the bloodstream into the inside of the cell. The cell uses glucose to generate energy. Without insulin, there can be plenty of sugar in your bloodstream but your cells are starving because they can't access it. It is interesting to note that brain cells and liver cells do not require insulin in order to absorb glucose from the bloodstream.

Type 1 diabetics cannot make enough insulin, therefore must inject it daily.

Type 2 diabetics usually have normal, or above normal levels of insulin in their bloodstream, but their cells no longer respond to the insulin. The different types of Diabetes will be described in more detail later on in this chapter.

Besides controlling your blood sugar level, insulin has a range of other metabolic effects in your body:

• Insulin stimulates the liver to store glucose in the form of glycogen

Much of the glucose that is absorbed from your small intestine after a meal travels straight to your liver where it is converted into glycogen for storage. Some glycogen is also stored in your muscles. People who have a fatty liver have a reduced capacity to store glycogen in their liver; therefore they convert more glucose into fat. Interestingly, the fitter you are, the better able your muscles are to store glycogen. Glycogen provides you with a quick source of energy when you need it.

• Insulin stimulates the liver to manufacture fatty acids

The body has a limited capacity to store glucose as glycogen, therefore when reserves are full the liver converts any excess glucose into fatty acids. The fatty acids are incorporated into lipoproteins, such as LDL and HDL cholesterol. Insulin particularly stimulates the liver to manufacture more LDL "bad" cholesterol. The fatty acids made by the liver can be stored within it (encouraging the development of fatty liver disease) and they are transported to fat cells (adipocytes) where they are converted into triglycerides; a storage form of fat. Therefore you can see that insulin stimulates your body to manufacture and store fat!

• Insulin inhibits the breakdown of body fat

It does this by inhibiting the enzyme in fat cells that is responsible for breaking down fat stores. In fact, insulin also enables glucose to enter fat cells, where it is converted into triglycerides. Therefore, insulin stimulates your fat cells to manufacture more fat, and inhibits the burning of body fat. Clearly you don't want large amounts of insulin in your body!

• Insulin increases water and salt retention

It also stimulates the growth of smooth muscle cells in artery walls. This promotes high blood pressure and also fluid retention.

• Insulin stimulates hunger

In particular it will make you hungry for high carbohydrate or high sugar foods.

• Insulin inhibits muscle growth

This is because it inhibits the release of growth hormone, which is needed for building new muscle mass. Growth hormone is also thought to delay the signs of aging.

Types of Diabetes

There are three main types of Diabetes:

- **Type 1 Diabetes:** This form of the disease occurs in ten to 15 percent of diabetics. It is an autoimmune disease that destroys the pancreas and renders it unable to produce sufficient amounts of insulin. Normally your immune system produces antibodies to fight off harmful bacteria and viruses; however in this case, antibodies are produced against the pancreas. Consequently, patients require daily insulin therapy in order to survive. The disease usually develops in childhood, before the age of 18 years, however it may occur in adulthood.

- **Type 2 Diabetes:** This is a much more common form of the disease, and accounts for 85 to 90 percent of all cases of Diabetes. In this instance, the body produces sufficient insulin, but the cells no longer respond to it properly. Syndrome X, (also known as insulin resistance) results in high blood insulin levels and it is a major forerunner to Type 2 Diabetes. Type 2 Diabetes was once called adult onset Diabetes because it predominantly occurred in people over the age of 40 years. However, that name has been dropped because the condition is now frequently diagnosed in childhood.

- **Gestational Diabetes:** This is a temporary form of Diabetes that occurs in three to eight percent of pregnant women who did not previously have Diabetes. The disease usually disappears after the baby is born, but women with the condition are at much greater risk of developing Type 2 Diabetes later in their life. Approximately 18 percent of pregnancies in the USA are affected by gestational Diabetes. The risk of gestational Diabetes is increased by being overweight, having a history of polycystic ovarian syndrome and having a family history of Type 2 Diabetes.

In most cases, gestational Diabetes is controlled by making improvements to the diet, such as avoiding sugar and eating less carbohydrate (grains, starches, cereals). If the Diabetes doesn't respond to these changes, the woman will have to inject insulin for the duration of the pregnancy. Poorly controlled gestational Diabetes increases the risk of giving birth to a large baby (possibly requiring a caesarian section) and makes a woman twice as likely to develop pre-eclampsia as other pregnant women.

There are a couple of other rare types of Diabetes that do not fit into any of these categories; they include genetic and drug related Diabetes, as well as Diabetes as a result of pancreatic disease.

How common is Diabetes?

Diabetes is the fastest growing chronic disease in the USA; in 2010 it was the seventh highest cause of death. In 2010 there were 18.8 million diabetics in the USA. It is also estimated that there were seven million undiagnosed diabetics. Many people do not realize they have Diabetes for some time before they are diagnosed; this is a problem because the high blood sugar could have already done considerable damage to their body.

The frightening fact is that more and more young children are being diagnosed with Type 2 Diabetes, when this used to be a disease of middle to old age. The main reason for this is the escalating rate of overweight and obesity in children. Weight gain around the abdominal area makes children more likely to develop Syndrome X, high blood sugar, as well as high cholesterol and blood pressure. This is a very disturbing trend because some children being diagnosed with Type 2 Diabetes are below the age of ten years. The incidence of Type 2 Diabetes in children is expected to escalate in the next decade, along with rates of overweight and obesity.

Incidence of Diabetes around the world

Diabetes is no longer a disease confined to wealthy developed nations. The World Health Organization estimates that by the year 2025, 80 percent of all new cases of Diabetes will occur in developing countries. Currently India has the world's highest diabetic population; there are 35 million diabetics living there, and in 20 years this figure is expected to grow to 75 million. Because Indians are so genetically susceptible to Type 2 Diabetes, they develop it at a much younger age than Caucasians; therefore suffer a lot more from its complications.

Rapid industrialization in India, China and other countries has allowed people living in cities to eat heavily processed, fast food and consequently develop the diseases common in developed nations. In some parts of Asia, Oceania, the Caribbean and the

Middle East, Diabetes affects between 12 and 20 percent of the adult population.[1] Poor access to medical care in developing nations means that Diabetes often goes undiagnosed, or is inadequately treated, therefore the complications and death rate are high.

Some nationalities are more prone to Diabetes than others; this is especially true for Asians. Chinese, Korean and Japanese people develop Type 2 Diabetes at a much lower body weight than Caucasians. This means they don't have to be very overweight to get the disease. Regardless of their weight, they are 60 percent more likely to develop Diabetes than Caucasians.

Worldwide, annual Diabetes deaths are approximately 3.8 million; this is equivalent to the global toll of HIV/AIDS and malaria combined![2]

2. Risk factors and symptoms of Diabetes

Risk factors for developing Type 2 Diabetes

This type of Diabetes is often referred to as a "lifestyle disease" because it is largely a result of obesity, lack of exercise and poor diet. It is true that 80 to 90 percent of type 2 diabetics are overweight or obese. If they were not overweight, they would probably not have developed the disease. Therefore, most of the risk factors that are described below relate in one way or another to being overweight. The great news is that the majority of these risk factors are under your control. If you reverse these factors, you have an excellent chance of reversing your Diabetes.

Here are the main risk factors for developing Type 2 Diabetes:

Obesity

Obesity is defined as being 20 percent or more above your ideal (what is considered healthy) body weight. Being ten percent above your ideal body weight categorizes you as overweight. There are a few ways of measuring whether your weight fits into the healthy category. The two most widely used methods are Body Mass Index (BMI) and waist to hip ratio.

• **Body Mass Index (BMI):** This is the most widely used method of assessing an individual's body weight. Having a Body Mass Index greater than 27 places you at increased risk of Type 2 Diabetes. You can work out your BMI by dividing your weight (in kilograms) by your height (in metres) squared.

For example, if you are 164cm tall and weigh 73 kilograms, you would work out your BMI as follows:

Body Mass Index = WEIGHT (kilograms)

HEIGHT X HEIGHT (meters)

For example, if you weigh 75 kilograms and are 1.69 meters tall, your BMI is:

$$\frac{75 \text{ kilograms}}{1.69 \times 1.69 \text{ meters}}$$

2.2 kilo = 1 lb
2.5cm = 1 inch
100 cm = 1 meter

BMI = 26

The table below will let you know how your weight is classified.

BMI Scale

Underweight	<18.5
Normal	19-25
Overweight	26-29
Obesity	30-39
Extreme obesity	>40

• **Waist to Hip Ratio:** BMI is not always the most reliable measure of obesity because some people with a lot of muscle on their body, or people with a large frame may be classed as overweight, when in fact their body fat percentage is low. Measuring your waist to hip ratio determines if you carry too much abdominal fat; fat stored here is more dangerous than fat located on other parts of your body. Having a large waist means you have a high amount of visceral fat in your body; this fat infiltrates and surrounds abdominal organs such as the liver, pancreas and heart. Excess weight on the thighs and buttocks is less of a health hazard because there are no important organs in that region of the body.

Some cultures, particularly Asians and Middle Eastern people may appear slim and fall into the "normal" category on the BMI scale, yet have an unfavorable waist to hip ratio and are at high risk of developing Type 2 Diabetes.

Instructions for calculating your waist to hip ratio:

While unclothed, stand up straight with your abdominal muscles relaxed. Using a tape measure, measure your waist at its narrowest part; this is usually an inch above the navel. Next measure your hips at their widest point. Now divide your waist measure by your hip measure. Anything above 0.80 for women and 0.90 for men reflects a greater risk of Type 2 Diabetes and cardiovascular disease.

For example, if your waist measures 37.4 inches (95cm) and your hips measure 35.43 inches (90cm), your waist to hip ratio is

$$\frac{37.4}{35.43} = 1.05$$ This figure indicates you are carrying too much weight over your abdominal area which is placing your health at risk.

How does obesity increase your risk of Type 2 Diabetes?

Fat cells secrete a number of different chemicals and hormones, especially fat cells around the abdomen. These chemicals have several biological actions that promote the development of Type 2 Diabetes:

- They reduce the effectiveness of insulin.
- Reduce the ability of your muscles to utilise glucose for energy.
- Increase the amount of glucose manufactured by your liver.
- Impair insulin release by the cells of your pancreas.

The more fat cells you have and the bigger they are, the more harmful chemicals and hormones they will release into your bloodstream. Therefore, being overweight makes it harder for your body to control your blood sugar level. This will almost inevitably make a person insulin resistant and cause them to develop Syndrome X.

• Syndrome X/Insulin Resistance

Syndrome X is a forerunner to Type 2 Diabetes. It is also known as metabolic syndrome, insulin resistance and impaired glucose tolerance. You are considered to have Syndrome X if you have central obesity, meaning you have a waist circumference greater than 31.5 inches (80cm) in European women and greater than 37 inches (94cm) in European men, plus two or more of the following four criteria:

• Elevated blood triglycerides: Greater than 149 mg/dL (1.69mmol/L).

• Low "good" HDL cholesterol: Less than 50 mg/dL (1.29mmol/L) in women and less than 40 mg/dL (1.04mmol/L) in men.

• High blood pressure: Greater than 130/85mm Hg

• Elevated fasting blood sugar: Greater than 99 mg/dL (5.5mmol/L)

Waist circumference measurements vary depending on ethnicity[3]; waist measurements that determine Syndrome X in Asians are as follows:

Chinese	waist >31.5 inches (80cm) in women
	waist >35.43 inches (90cm) in men
South Asians (Malay and Asian-Indian)	waist >31.5 inches (80cm) in women
	waist >35.43 inches (90cm) in men
Japanese	waist >35.43 inches (90cm) in women
	waist >33.46 inches (85cm) in men

The prevalence of Syndrome X is rapidly increasing across all age groups, and many people with Syndrome X go on to develop Type 2 Diabetes. Research has shown that approximately 50% of men and women over the age of 50 have Syndrome X. It is also very prevalent in overweight children.

How does Syndrome X increase your risk of Type 2 Diabetes?

Syndrome X is marked by elevated blood levels of the hormone insulin. Insulin is a hormone that enables glucose to enter cells, where it is used for energy. Insulin resistance occurs when the cells of your body no longer respond to normal levels of insulin, therefore the pancreas secretes ever increasing quantities of insulin. As insulin becomes less and less effective, blood glucose levels start to rise. High insulin levels have a number of harmful effects in the body, as described in Chapter One. In particular, insulin stimulates the creation of more body fat, particularly around the waist. Fat gain here worsens insulin resistance, which further promotes a rise in blood glucose levels.

Studies have shown that healthy people secrete an average of 31 units of insulin daily, while obese type 2 diabetics secrete approximately 114 units of insulin daily.[4]

- **Losing weight is the key to reversing Syndrome X and preventing Type 2 Diabetes in the first place**

Once the fasting blood sugar level gets above 5.5mmol/L, we can say a person has pre-Diabetes, meaning if they continue with their current diet and lifestyle, they are very likely to develop Type 2 Diabetes in the next five years. It is interesting to realize that even if your blood sugar never gets to diabetic levels (6.9mmol/L fasting), you are still at increased risk of some of the complications of Diabetes because high blood sugar has a number of toxic effects. It is estimated that one in four people have insulin resistance. Insulin resistance is a lot easier to reverse than Type 2 Diabetes; by following our recommendations that begin in Chapter Six, you can easily reverse this condition and lose weight.

The risk factors for developing Syndrome X are much the same as those for Type 2 Diabetes, including being overweight, having a diet high in refined carbohydrates and trans fats, lack of exercise and genetic factors.

Even if they never go on to develop Type 2 Diabetes, people with Syndrome X are three times more likely to have a heart attack or stroke than people without this condition, and twice as likely to die from a heart attack or stroke.

• Lack of exercise

Lack of exercise is one of the most important factors implicated in the cause of Syndrome X and Type 2 Diabetes. The average person's diet is becoming richer in calories, fat and carbohydrate, yet no exercise is done to burn off the excess calories. Regular exercise helps to keep you in a healthy weight range and it increases motivation to follow a healthy diet. Regular exercise also helps to keep your blood sugar in the normal range and it improves your body's sensitivity to insulin. Exercise really is medicine; it has so many beneficial effects on your metabolism. The importance of exercise will be covered in detail in Chapter Eight.

• Poor diet

People often ask the question "does eating sugar cause Diabetes?" The answer is yes it can, but it's not the only factor when it comes to diet. Sugar, as well as high carbohydrate foods like bread, pasta, rice, potatoes, breakfast cereals and any food that contains flour are digested into glucose and they raise your blood sugar and insulin levels when you eat them. They also cause a rise in your triglyceride level. If you eat a lot of these foods, and you don't exercise and you are genetically susceptible, they can cause you to gain weight, develop Syndrome X and then Type 2 Diabetes. Eating a lot of junk food and highly processed food, along with not eating fresh vegetables can also make you overweight and more likely to develop Type 2 Diabetes. Eating more food than you need and not burning off the excess calories through exercise can make you overweight and place you at increased risk of Type 2 Diabetes.

● The specific dietary habits that place you at increased risk of Type 2 Diabetes are:

● **Consuming too much carbohydrate** – Grains, starches and sugar make up a great deal of the average person's diet now. It is common to eat breakfast cereal or toast for breakfast, a sandwich for lunch and pasta, rice or potatoes for dinner. In between meals, cookies and coffee or tea containing sugar contribute even more carbohydrate to the diet. To make things worse, the carbohydrates many people eat are refined and stripped of nutrients; for example white bread, white rice and foods made of white flour. This means the diet contains a lot of high glycemic index carbohydrates, which makes blood sugar levels rise rapidly and promotes high insulin levels. The glycemic index is described in detail in Chapter Six. Some people are more sensitive to a high carbohydrate diet than others and gain weight more easily eating a lot of these foods.

Consuming too much sugar is very easy to do. Sugar is in so many foods that people eat each day, without even realizing it. Many breakfast cereals, pasta sauces, bread, simmer sauces and numerous other foods contain added sugar. Soda pop consumption has rapidly increased among children and teenagers. Fruit juice, cordial, sports drinks and energy drinks all add even more sugar to the average person's diet.

● **Not eating enough fiber.** Fiber slows down the absorption of nutrients in the intestinal tract, including glucose. Therefore fiber in a meal lowers the glycemic index of a meal by slowing down the rise in blood sugar that occurs after eating carbohydrates. Fiber is found in all vegetables, fruit, nuts and seeds (such as almonds, walnuts, hazelnuts, sunflower seeds and others), legumes (such as kidney beans, borlotti beans, lentils and others) and grains such as brown rice, oats and rye bread. Beware of highly processed, sugar containing breakfast cereals that claim to be high in fiber; they are usually also high in sugar. It is preferable to obtain fiber in your diet through natural, unprocessed foods such as those listed above.

There are two main types of fiber: soluble fiber and insoluble fiber. Water soluble fiber has more benefits for blood sugar control; it is found primarily in fruits, vegetables, flaxseeds, psyllium, oats, barley, beans, peas and lentils. This type of fiber forms a gel-like consistency in the intestinal tract, which slows the absorption of nutrients, including glucose.

• **Eating the wrong fats** – The types of fat you eat play an important role in your risk of Type 2 Diabetes. Remember that insulin must communicate with receptors on your cell membranes in order to allow glucose to enter your cells. Cell membranes are predominantly made of fatty acids. Therefore the types of fat you eat influence the health and function of your cell membranes. Having trans fatty acids in your cell membranes reduces the ability of insulin to bind to receptors on your cells, fostering the development of insulin resistance. Trans fatty acids are an unnatural fat found in many margarines, cooking oils and foods containing these, such as cookies, crackers, donuts, cakes, fast food and fried food. They are commonly used in processed food because they are cheap and have a long shelf life. There is more information about trans fatty acids in Chapter Six.

Not having enough omega 3 fatty acids in your diet also impairs the ability of insulin to function. Clinical studies have shown that monounsaturated fats and omega 3 fats improve insulin action.[5] Anything that improves insulin action helps to prevent Syndrome X and Type 2 Diabetes. Monounsaturated fats are found in olive oil, macadamias, almonds, Brazil nuts, avocados and sesame seeds. Omega 3 fats are found mainly in fish and other seafood, and also in flaxseeds, walnuts and green leafy vegetables. There is more information about all types of fats in Chapter Six.

• **Mineral and antioxidant deficiencies**. People who develop insulin resistance and Type 2 Diabetes are more likely to be deficient in certain nutrients. These deficiencies can inhibit insulin from working efficiently; therefore greater amounts of insulin must be secreted by the pancreas. The most common mineral deficiencies linked to Type 2 Diabetes are:

• Chromium

Chromium helps your cells to communicate more efficiently with insulin, thereby helping to prevent high blood insulin levels. People who are deficient in chromium are more likely to experience sugar and carbohydrate cravings, Hypoglycemia and to develop Type 2

Diabetes. It is hard to get enough chromium through your diet; the richest sources are brewer's yeast and liver. If you have Type 2 Diabetes it is very beneficial to take a chromium supplement.

• Magnesium

Research has shown that people with a high magnesium intake are less likely to develop Type 2 Diabetes, and diabetics tend to have lower magnesium stores. Magnesium helps to increase your body's sensitivity to insulin. Many people are magnesium deficient because they do not eat enough vegetables, nuts, seeds and whole grains; all rich sources of magnesium. Processed food like white flour products are largely stripped of magnesium.

A lack of antioxidants in your diet also increases the risk of Diabetes. Antioxidants help to protect the fatty acids in your cell membranes from damage incurred by free radicals. Free radicals are highly reactive molecules, generated through normal metabolism as well as pollution, cigarettes, radiation, stress and other factors. They are capable of damaging cell membranes, therefore impairing the ability of insulin to communicate with your cells. Antioxidants help to keep insulin receptors on your cells healthy. Good sources of antioxidants include vegetables, fruit, green tea, raw nuts and seeds, red wine and dark chocolate. The effects of minerals and antioxidants on Diabetes is discussed in greater detail in Chapter Nine.

• **Eating barbecued, toasted and caramelized foods.** When food undergoes one of these processes, a reaction between sugar and protein forms what are known as glycated (or glycosylated) end products. Eating foods containing glycated end products increases the risk of developing Type 2 Diabetes and heart disease. This same reaction between sugar and protein can also occur inside your body if you have high blood sugar and it increases your rate of aging. You can read about glycated end products in Chapter Four.

• Family history

There is definitely a genetic component in Type 2 Diabetes. Having a family history of Type 2 Diabetes significantly increases your chance of developing the disease; this is especially so if it is a parent or sibling. In the case of identical twins, if one twin develops the disease, the other twin has a 70 to 90 percent chance of becoming a type 2 diabetic. If both of your parents have Type 2 Diabetes, your risk of developing the disease is greater than 40 percent.[6]

People are now being diagnosed with Type 2 Diabetes earlier in life, so if your parent was diagnosed with the disease when they were in their sixties, you could develop the disease in your forties or earlier. Women who had gestational Diabetes while pregnant are at greater risk of developing full blown Type 2 Diabetes. Having a family history of Diabetes doesn't guarantee that you will develop it; if you avoid becoming overweight, exercise and eat well, you can avoid it entirely.

• Ethnic background

Some nationalities are far more likely to develop Type 2 Diabetes than others. People with Australian Aboriginal, Hispanic, African, Pacific Island or Asian ancestry are between two and six times more prone to the disease than Caucasians. Type 2 Diabetes is an enormous problem among Australian Aborigines and Torres Strait Island populations; the disease affects one in four indigenous Australians and is increasingly being diagnosed in children as young as ten. An article appearing in *The Australian* newspaper in November 2006, quoted Diabetes expert Professor Zimmet as saying "Without urgent action there certainly is a real risk of a major wipe-out of indigenous communities, if not total extinction, within this century,".[7] Diabetes was never a problem centuries ago when Aborigines followed their traditional diet and lifestyle. However, high carbohydrate foods like bread, pasta, soda pops, cookies and alcohol were not a part of traditional cuisine; their introduction into a population at great genetic risk of Diabetes has proven disastrous.

Another population very susceptible to Diabetes is the Pima Indians of Arizona; they actually have the highest rate of obesity and Type 2 Diabetes anywhere in the world. Research has shown that these people also have a strong genetic predisposition to Diabetes, but diet and lifestyle are playing a greater part. We know this because Pima Indians who live in Mexico and still follow a traditional diet and lifestyle have a very low rate of obesity and Type 2 Diabetes. In Pima Indians who live in Arizona and follow a typical American diet, the obesity rate is 70 percent and the rate of Type 2 Diabetes is 22 percent. Pima Indians who live in Mexico still cultivate traditional crops such as beans, corn, potatoes and seasonal vegetables and fruit such as apples, peaches, bell pepper, tomatoes and zucchini. Only ten percent of these people are obese, and Type 2 Diabetes is a rarity.

• Medication use

It is known that several medications can hasten the development of Syndrome X and Type 2 Diabetes in susceptible people. These medications include:

• Thiazide diuretics (fluid tablets) and beta blockers, which slow down the heart rate and are used in high blood pressure and angina.

• The oral contraceptive pill, especially those containing the progestagens levo-norgestrel or norethisterone.

• Steroids, such as cortisone and body building hormones.

• Zyprexa, a mood stabilizer that is used for schizophrenia, bipolar disorder and related conditions.

Symptoms of Diabetes

Both type 1 and Type 2 Diabetes can produce the same symptoms, but symptoms are usually a lot more obvious in type 1 Diabetes. This means it is generally diagnosed faster. The symptoms of Type 2 Diabetes can be very mild and some people get no symptoms at all until their Diabetes is at an advanced stage and irreversible damage has been done to their body. The earlier Diabetes is detected and treated, the better chance you have of avoiding the complications of the disease. The following are all possible symptoms of Diabetes:

• Increased hunger

• Increased thirst

• Fatigue

• Increased urination, particularly at night

- Sores that do not heal
- Infections such as thrush or skin infections such as boils or fungal skin infections
- Blurred vision
- Burning, numbness or tingling in the feet or hands
- Weight loss or weight gain
- Irritability and mood changes
- Headaches
- Dizziness
- Erectile dysfunction
- Bell's palsy and carpal tunnel syndrome. These conditions can both be a result of nerve damage caused by episodes of high blood sugar.

Often people with type 1 Diabetes are of normal weight or underweight, and people with Type 2 Diabetes are usually overweight.

Skin signs of Syndrome X and Type 2 Diabetes

The following skin signs are usually present in people with Diabetes, or people at high risk of developing it:

• Skin tags

These are very common in overweight people and typically develop on the neck, armpits, eyelids and groin regions. They are a piece of skin that projects from the surrounding skin and may be smooth, irregular, flesh colored or darker. Skin tags can be simply raised above the skin or they can be attached by a stalk. Skin tags are a good indicator that you are suffering from Syndrome X and probably have a high triglyceride and/or low HDL cholesterol level. You can see what skin tags look like by visiting the following website: http://dermatology.cdlib.org/95/pearls/tags/2.jpg

• Acanthosis nigricans

This is a thickened, darkened area of skin commonly found on skin folds. It usually occurs on the back of the neck, under the arms, under the breasts, at the belt line and in the groin. The skin can look brown and leathery. The condition is commonly found in people who are overweight, have Type 2 Diabetes or polycystic ovarian syndrome. You can see what acanthosis nigricans looks like by visiting the following website: http://dermatology.cdlib.org/DOJvol6num1/original/acanthosis/figure02b.jpg

3. Tests to diagnose and monitor Diabetes

Essential tests for diabetics

This section will cover the standard tests done to detect Type 2 Diabetes, as well as the ongoing tests required to monitor this condition.

Who should be tested for Diabetes?

We recommend that everyone who fits into a category below has a blood test for Type 2 Diabetes:

- People over 45 years of age who are overweight
- People over 45 years of age who have high blood pressure
- People over 45 years of age who have one or more family members with Diabetes
- Everyone over 55 years of age
- People who have heart disease or have had a heart attack
- Women who currently have polycystic ovarian syndrome, or have had it in the past
- Women who have had gestational Diabetes (high blood sugar while pregnant)
- People who have been diagnosed with Syndrome X, insulin resistance or impaired glucose tolerance
- People over 35 years of age who are Aboriginal or a Torres Strait Islander
- People over 35 years of age who are a Pacific Islander, Chinese, Indian or African American
- Men over 45 years of age with erectile dysfunction

If you fall into one of these groups you are considered at high risk for developing Type 2 Diabetes.

Blood tests to diagnose Type 2 Diabetes

The following test is used to diagnose Type 2 Diabetes:

Fasting blood glucose: This test is performed after you have fasted for 12 hours, therefore early in the morning before breakfast is usually most convenient. A healthy blood sugar level is between 64 and 97 mg/dL (3.6 and 5.4mmol/L). If your blood sugar is between 99 and 124 mg/dL (5.5 and 6.9mmol/L) you are considered to have impaired glucose tolerance, also known as pre-Diabetes. A fasting blood sugar level of 124mg/dL (6.9 mmol/L) or above indicates Diabetes.

Please note this test is usually performed on two separate occasions, to confirm the diagnosis.

All diabetics should have a fasting blood sugar test performed by their doctor every six months.

Sometimes a **random blood glucose** test is done; this means you haven't fasted for 12 hours prior to having the blood test. A healthy random blood glucose level is between 64 and 138 mg/dL (3.6mmol/L and 7.7mmol/L). If your random blood glucose is 198 mg/dL (11mmol/L) or higher, on two separate occasions, you likely have Diabetes.

If the blood sugar level is higher than normal, but not high enough to be considered diabetic, a glucose tolerance test is usually performed.

Factors that can affect your blood sugar level

Things that can lower your blood sugar include:

- Fasting

- Exercise

- After administering an insulin injection (if you are on insulin therapy)

Things that can raise your blood sugar include:

- Eating
- Illness, such as an infection
- Stress

Glucose tolerance test:

If your blood sugar level is higher than ideal, but not high enough to be considered diabetic, you will usually be asked to have a glucose tolerance test. This measures your blood sugar level after you ingest a test dose of glucose (2.6 ounces, or 75 grams). Your blood sugar is tested over a period of two hours or (ideally) longer. It is best if your insulin levels are also tested along with glucose, therefore making this a glucose insulin tolerance test.

The normal values for a glucose tolerance test are below:

Time	Normal	Impaired glucose tolerance	Diabetes
Fasting	glucose 3.6-5.4mmol/L Insulin below 10mU/L	glucose 5.5-6.9mmol/L insulin above 10mU/L	glucose >6.9mmol/L
2 hour	glucose less than 7.1mmol/L Insulin 5-50mU/L	glucose 7.2-11.0mmol/L insulin above 50mU/L	glucose above 11mmol/L

What does the test involve?

For three days before having a glucose tolerance test you are required to follow a high carbohydrate diet, consuming approximately 150 grams of carbohydrate each day. This means eating toast or cereal for breakfast, a sandwich for lunch and pasta or rice for dinner, or similar. You are required to fast for approximately 12 hours before having this test, but do not fast for more than 16 hours. Don't consume any caffeinated beverages such as tea or coffee before the test because they can alter the results.

At the start of the glucose tolerance test your blood sugar will be tested and after that you will be given a sweet liquid to drink, which contains 2.6 ounces (75 grams) of glucose. Your blood sugar level will be tested again two hours later.

In some circumstances a glucose tolerance test should NOT be performed; these include:

- When you are ill; for example during an infection, recently after surgery or trauma.

- If you are known to have Diabetes.

- If you take certain medications, including corticosteroids and beta adrenergic agonists (some drugs used in the treatment of asthma). These drugs can make the results of the test unreliable.

Whatever happened to urine tests for Diabetes?

Until the mid 1970s, the only way diabetics could check their blood sugar was indirectly, through checking the amount of glucose in their urine. Normally the kidneys reabsorb glucose from the blood that they continually filter. However, if the blood sugar gets too high, the kidneys can't reabsorb all the glucose and some spills over into the urine.

In general, glucose will start to appear in your urine when your blood sugar level reaches 180 mg/dL (10mmol/L) or more. If your blood sugar is lower than 180 mg/dL (10mmol/L), your urine will not contain glucose. As you can see, this testing method is very insensitive, and a blood sugar reading much lower than 180 mg/dL (10mmol/L) is still very dangerous and can cause diabetic complications.

> **In summary, you are considered to have Type 2 Diabetes if you meet one of these criteria:**
>
> - Fasting blood sugar higher than 124 mg/dL (6.9mmol/L)
> - A random blood glucose (non-fasting) level greater than 198 mg/dL (11mmol/L)
> - A glucose tolerance test showing a two hour blood glucose level greater than 198 mg/dL (11mmol/L)

Diagnosis of Gestational Diabetes

Gestational Diabetes typically starts in the 24th to 28th week of pregnancy. The test used to diagnose gestational Diabetes is called a glucose challenge test. It involves drinking a 1.8 ounce (50 gram) glucose solution and having a blood test one hour later. A blood sugar level above 140 mg/dL (7.8mmol/L) may indicate gestational Diabetes. If the blood sugar level is borderline, the patient has a glucose tolerance test on another day to confirm the diagnosis. The glucose challenge test is not a fasting test.

A pregnant woman is considered to have gestational Diabetes if her fasting blood glucose level is greater than 99 mg/dL (5.5mmol/L) or her two hour glucose tolerance test reveals a blood sugar level greater than 144 mg/dL (8mmol/L).

Essential ongoing tests to monitor Diabetes

The closer to normal your blood sugar level is, the less likely you are to experience diabetic complications. The tests described in this section of the book will help you to keep a close eye on your blood sugar and other markers that diabetics need to be aware of. By regularly monitoring your Diabetes, you can check the effects any diet, supplement and lifestyle changes are having on your condition.

- **Glycosylated hemoglobin** (HbA1c): Also called glycated hemoglobin, this test determines the average amount of glucose that has been present in your bloodstream for the previous three months. Specifically this test measures the amount of glucose that has been bound to the hemoglobin in your red blood cells; your red blood cells live for approximately three months. Glycosylated means sugar coated; this test literally measures how much sugar is coating the hemoglobin in your red blood cells. A normal HbA1c level for diabetics is 3.5-6.0%. A level greater than 7% indicates poor blood sugar control and greater risk of developing diabetic complications. You should aim for an HbA1c of less than 5.5%. All diabetics should have an HbA1c test done every six months.

• **Fasting insulin:** This test can reveal the degree of insulin resistance (Syndrome X) a person has. High fasting insulin levels are a feature of Syndrome X and Type 2 Diabetes. Normal fasting insulin is between 4 and 10 mU/L. Results above 10 indicate insulin resistance. A very low fasting insulin level in a type 2 diabetic can indicate pancreatic failure, whereby the pancreas is no longer able to manufacture sufficient insulin. A C-peptide test is recommended in that instance.

• **Fructosamine:** This blood test is not used often and is unnecessary in most cases. It measures the blood sugar level over the previous three weeks.

• **C-peptide:** This test can determine how much insulin a person is producing and whether insulin therapy is appropriate for a diabetic. The pancreas produces a large protein called pro-insulin. A fraction of this protein (C-peptide) is cut off by enzymes and the C-peptide plus insulin are both secreted into the bloodstream. Insulin that has been injected into the body has no C-peptide.

Measuring C-peptide levels tells us the degree of pancreatic function in a diabetic. Type 2 diabetics start out with high blood insulin levels that their body is no longer responding to. However, over time a diabetic may develop what is known as pancreatic burn out, whereby the pancreatic cells are worn out and are no longer able to manufacture insulin.

If C-peptide levels are normal or high, we know that a type 2 diabetic can still manufacture insulin. Very low C-peptide levels indicate that a type 2 diabetic will need to start insulin therapy in order to control their blood sugar.

If you have been diagnosed with Diabetes, your doctor will usually order a range of additional tests to check if you have developed any diabetic complications yet. Because diabetics are more prone to a range of other health problems, such as heart attacks and strokes, your doctor will want to evaluate your risk factors for these as well.

Other important tests for diabetics

• Blood pressure

More than half of all type 1 and type 2 diabetics have high blood pressure; this places them at significantly increased risk of heart attacks, strokes and kidney damage. Keeping your blood pressure in the normal range can help to protect you from developing these conditions. Ideal blood pressure is around 120/80. It is important to not let your blood pressure get greater than 130/85.

Our recommendations for reversing Diabetes that begin in Chapter Six will also help to keep your blood pressure healthy. If that is not successful, you may need medication to control your blood pressure. Your blood pressure should be checked every six months by your doctor when you visit him or her for your Diabetes blood tests. If your blood pressure always rises in your doctor's surgery, you may want to buy a blood pressure monitor to use at home. That way you can test your blood pressure in a relaxed, stress free environment.

• Cholesterol and other blood fats

Elevated cholesterol and triglycerides are very common in diabetics and may place them at increased risk of heart attacks and strokes. Commonly diabetics have high levels of LDL "bad" cholesterol and triglycerides and low levels of HDL "good" cholesterol. These are common features of Syndrome X, or insulin resistance and are often present long before the Diabetes develops. Diabetics often have high blood levels of high sensitivity C-reactive protein. This is a protein made in the liver which is associated with high levels of inflammation in the body. Inflammation is an initiating factor in the development of cardiovascular disease and other serious diseases.

The following table lists the normal levels of blood fats you should aim for:

Blood fat	Normal Reference Range
Total cholesterol	150 - 212 mg/dL (3.9-5.5 mmol/L)
HDL cholesterol	34 - 81 mg/dL (0.9-2.1 mmol/L)
LDL cholesterol	65 - 135 mg/dL (1.7-3.5 mmol/L)
Triglycerides	44 - 149 mg/dL (0.5-1.69 mmol/L)

High sensitivity C-reactive protein should be less than 3mg/L

Following our diet recommendations in Chapter Six will help to reduce your risk of cardiovascular disease. For more comprehensive information about reducing your risk of cardiovascular disease see our book *Cholesterol the Real Truth*.

• Kidney function test

Diabetes is the most common cause of kidney failure, dialysis and kidney transplant.[8] Regular monitoring of kidney function can detect problems at the earliest stage, therefore greatly reducing the risk of end stage kidney disease. Every six months you should have a urine test checking for the presence of albumin and a blood test checking your creatinine levels.

Albumin is a type of protein; if it is present in your urine it usually means your kidneys are starting to become damaged and are leaky. It is an early warning sign of diabetic kidney disease (also called nephropathy).

A normal level of albumin in the urine is less than 30mg albumin/g creatinine.

For an accurate reading, you should avoid strenuous exercise for 24 hours before having this test.

Creatinine is a waste product of protein digestion that is normally filtered by the kidneys.

- Normal blood creatinine levels for an adult female are 0.05-0.11mmol/L.

- Normal blood creatinine levels for an adult male are 0.06-0.12mmol/L.

High blood levels of creatinine can indicate impaired filtration by the kidneys.

- Eye exam

Diabetes is the leading cause of blindness in people over the age of 60. Once a year every diabetic should see an eye specialist (ophthalmologist) for a retinal eye exam. The doctor will insert eye drops that dilate your pupil so that he or she can get a better view of your retina (the back part of your eyes). Your eyes should also be checked for cataracts and glaucoma.

- Foot exam

Every six months when you see your doctor for blood tests, you should also have a foot inspection. Your doctor will check for any lesions or ulcers, abnormalities in your nails and the quality of your circulation. You should also have a sensory test to make sure there is no nerve damage in your feet. Diabetics are very prone to foot problems for several reasons and Diabetes is unfortunately a common cause of non-trauma related amputations.

- Dental checkup

Ideally everyone should visit a dentist every six months. Diabetics are more prone to tooth and gum problems than the general population.

- Urine ketone testing

Diabetics can check for the presence of ketones in their urine at home using testing strips available from a pharmacy. This test is mostly used by insulin dependant diabetics or diabetics with difficult to control, consistently high blood sugar. Dangerously high levels of ketones will appear in the urine when there is insufficient insulin available. This means the body cannot use glucose for energy, therefore burns body fat stores instead.

This condition is called diabetic ketoacidosis and is accompanied by extremely high blood sugar levels and can cause severe dehydration. Urine ketone testing is only required for type 1 diabetics or any diabetic with poorly controlled blood sugar. Ketoacidosis is most likely to occur when a diabetic is sick or injured. If your blood sugar level is unusually high and you don't know the reason, you should check your urinary ketone level.

Checking your blood sugar level yourself at home

It is important to regularly check your blood sugar level yourself at home. This way you will have greater control of your Diabetes and know which factors have a positive and negative effect on your blood sugar. It is especially important to check your blood sugar level if you feel unwell and when you make changes to your diet, exercise level and lifestyle habits. A significant study called the United Kingdom Prospective Diabetes Study (UKPDS) found that diabetics who keep a close eye on their blood sugar level are much less likely to develop diabetic complications and enjoy much better health than diabetics who don't regularly check their blood sugar.

When is the best time to check your blood sugar?

The best time to check your blood glucose level is after you wake and before breakfast, two hours after eating and at bedtime. If you have good control of your blood sugar level and your diet and routine are consistent, it is fine to just check your blood sugar on waking only.

Summary of essential tests for diabetics

TEST	WHY IT'S IMPORTANT	FREQUENCY	IDEAL RANGE
Fasting blood glucose level	This is an indicator of how well your Diabetes is being managed and a reflection of your diet.	You should test this at least once daily, such as before breakfast. Your GP should do this test at least every 6 months.	Aim for fasting glucose level below 5.5 mmol/L.
HbA$_{1c}$	Indicates your average blood sugar level over the previous 3 months. The higher this figure, the more likely you are to suffer the complications of Diabetes.	Tested every 3 months if your Diabetes is poorly controlled; tested every 6 months if well controlled.	Between 3.5 and 6% is considered normal for diabetics. Aim for less than 5.5%.
Blood pressure	Many diabetics develop high blood pressure; this places them at increased risk of stroke, heart attacks and kidney failure.	Every 6 months.	Ideally 120/80 and no higher than 130/85.

Blood lipids (fats)	Diabetics are at increased risk of cardiovascular disease.	Every 6 months.	Total cholesterol 3.9-5.5mmol/L HDL cholesterol 0.9-2.1mmol/L LDL cholesterol 1.7-3.5mmol/L Triglycerides 0.5-1.69mmol/L
Kidney function	Diabetes is the most common cause of kidney failure. The earlier an abnormality is detected, the less likely end stage kidney disease will occur.	Every 6 months.	Urinary albumin should be less than 30mg albumin/g creatinine. Blood creatinine should be 0.05-0.11mmol/L for females and 0.06-0.12mmol/L for males.
Eye exam	Diabetics are prone to developing several eye diseases which can result in loss of sight.	Every 12 months.	An eye specialist (ophthalmologist) will perform several tests.

Foot exam	Damage to nerves and blood vessels makes diabetics more prone to foot problems that can lead to several complications, including amputations.	You should check your feet daily for any sores, numbness, pain or other abnormalities. Your GP should perform a thorough foot exam every 6 months, including checking for nerve damage.	Any sores or infections should be treated promptly to avoid complications such as ulcers.
Dental exam	Diabetics are more prone to tooth and gum disease.	A visit to the dentist every 6 months.	Any problems or infections should be treated promptly.
Fasting insulin level	This is an indicator of how insulin resistant you are. Insulin levels rise with weight gain and this will make blood sugar harder to control.	Every 12 months.	Fasting insulin should be between 4 and 10 mU/L.

4. The health complications of Diabetes

Diabetes is a terrible disease; it can greatly reduce the quality of your life, make you more prone to several serious diseases and cut your life short prematurely. There are both short term and long term complications of Diabetes. Short term complications such as Hypoglycemia (low blood sugar), Hyperglycemia (high blood sugar) and diabetic ketoacidosis are more common in type 1 diabetics.

High blood sugar over a sustained period of time has many detrimental health consequences, therefore the longer a person has Diabetes, the worse the health consequences. Diabetes causes damage to the small and large blood vessels of the body, impairing circulation and the delivery of oxygen and nutrients to tissues. Diabetes also causes nerve damage. Damage to nerves and blood vessels is the major factor responsible for the long term complications of Diabetes. The long term complications of type 1 and Type 2 Diabetes are the same.

The main complications of Diabetes are:

• Heart disease

Four out of five people with Diabetes die of heart disease.[9] Diabetes is the biggest risk factor for heart disease; other risk factors include high blood pressure, obesity, smoking, high triglycerides and low levels of HDL "good" cholesterol. The more of these risk factors you have, the greater your chance of developing heart disease.

Diabetics are very prone to developing atherosclerosis; this is where fatty plaques form in blood vessels, particularly the arteries that supply the heart and brain with blood. Sugar is sticky and having high blood sugar levels means the blood is more likely to form clots that can block blood vessels. People with Diabetes are also more likely to develop heart failure; this is where the heart is not able to pump blood adequately. This can cause fluid build-up in the lungs, producing difficulty breathing and fluid retention in other parts of the body, particularly the legs.

High blood sugar can damage the nerves that regulate the heart beat. This can eventually cause an out of rhythm condition of the heart called arrhythmia. As fasting blood sugar rises, so too does the risk of heart disease. Studies have shown that even people who are not considered diabetic still run a much higher risk of heart disease if their blood sugar is higher than ideal.[10, 11]

Diabetics are also more likely to have blood vessels that are clogged with fatty plaques in their legs. This is called peripheral vascular disease and can produce the following symptoms:

- Cramps in your legs while you walk. This is called intermittent claudication.

- Cold feet.

- Loss of hair on the lower parts of the legs.

- Reduced or absent pulses on the lower legs or feet.

• Stroke

The brain has a vast network of blood vessels that supply it with oxygen rich blood. A stroke occurs when one of the blood vessels is blocked or damaged, so that oxygen cannot reach a part of the brain. There are two types of strokes:

- Ischemic strokes are caused by a blockage of an artery, such as from a blood clot or fatty plaque.

- Hemorrhagic strokes are caused by rupture of an artery.

If a region of the brain is deprived of oxygen for more than four minutes, the brain tissue will start to die. People with Diabetes are at increased risk of stroke even if they don't have other risk factors such as high blood pressure, obesity and cigarette smoking. Diabetics who have a stroke fare worse than people who don't have Diabetes.

• Eye damage

People with Diabetes are prone to three types of eye diseases: retinopathy, cataracts and glaucoma. However, short term very high blood sugar can cause temporary blurred vision and this can be restored when blood sugar is returned to a lower level. High blood glucose levels cause the lens in your eye to swell and this affects your ability to see. Your vision should return to normal after your blood sugar is controlled; although this can take up to three months.

The more serious eye problems diabetics are susceptible to include:

• **Retinopathy**: The retina is a collection of light sensitive cells at the back of each eye. In diabetics the retina can get damaged from several tiny hemorrhages, scarring, damaged tiny blood vessels and the attachment of glucose molecules from the bloodstream to proteins in the retina. The attachment of glucose to proteins in the body is called glycosylation and is discussed in more detail later on in this chapter. Research has shown that 20 years after being diagnosed with Diabetes, 80 percent of type 1 diabetics and 20 percent of type 2 diabetics have some degree of retinopathy. In the United States it is the leading cause of blindness in people over the age of 60 years. The better control you have over your blood sugar, the less likely you are to develop retinopathy. It is also essential to have plenty of antioxidants in your diet, as they help to protect your retina.

• **Cataracts**: A cataract is a fogging or clouding over of the lens of the eye. The lens allows you to see and focus on objects. The risk of cataracts increases with age. Around 2.5 percent of people in their forties have cataracts and 99 percent of people in their nineties. Diabetics tend to get cataracts earlier in life and they progress faster than in non-diabetics. This is because of the damage glucose does to the proteins in the lens. Cataracts produce blurred or glared vision and if severe, surgery may be required to remove the lens and insert an implant. Free radical damage to the lens is a leading cause of cataracts; this just highlights the greatly increased need diabetics have for antioxidants.

• **Glaucoma**: This condition results from a build up of pressure inside the eye, meaning that fluid inside the eye cannot drain properly. The increased pressure damages nerves and blood vessels in the eye, compromising vision. In most cases glaucoma doesn't cause any symptoms until the condition is advanced and vision becomes severely impaired. In some cases glaucoma can cause blurred vision, watery eyes, seeing a halo around lights, headaches or aching eyes. All diabetics should have a test for glaucoma by an eye doctor each year. The earlier glaucoma is detected the better the outcome.

• Kidney disease (nephropathy)

Diabetes is the biggest cause of kidney failure. Nearly a third of people with Diabetes develop kidney disease. Your kidneys function to remove waste products and excess water from the bloodstream, which are released as urine. The kidneys are comprised of a system of tubes and blood vessels called nephrons. That's why disease of the nephrons is called nephropathy. The main structure in the nephron is a group of closely woven blood vessels called the glomerulus, which acts as a filter.

High blood sugar and high blood pressure cause damage to the glomerulus and make the tiny blood vessels leaky. People with Diabetes also usually have blood vessels that are clogged with fat (atherosclerosis), impairing circulation and further increasing the risk of kidney disease. If the glomerulus has been damaged, protein will leak from the bloodstream and be lost in the urine. This protein is called albumin and its presence in urine is called microalbuminurea. If enough glomeruli have been damaged, the kidneys cannot function properly and the patient is said to have kidney failure. If this is severe enough, the patient may require dialysis and then a kidney transplant.

People with Diabetes are also more likely to have related problems like repeated bladder infections and damage to the nerves that travel to the bladder. This can cause symptoms such as urinary urgency, frequency, incontinence and needing to urinate frequently at night. Diabetics are also at greater risk of developing kidney stones, particularly uric acid kidney stones because they have very acidic urine. Obesity and Syndrome X are also associated with more acidic urine.

In people with Type 2 Diabetes, there is often some degree of kidney damage when they are diagnosed. This is because high blood sugar, high blood pressure and atherosclerosis are usually present for some time before the official diagnosis of Diabetes is made. Mild to moderate kidney disease usually doesn't cause any symptoms at all, however the following symptoms are possible:

- Weight gain

- Swelling of the face, feet and hands

- Muscle twitching

- Abnormalities in the heart's rhythm (this is because of high levels of potassium in the bloodstream)

If kidney disease becomes more severe, the kidneys cannot remove waste from the bloodstream. A high level of toxins in the bloodstream is called uraemia. It causes people to be confused, disoriented or comatose.

Kidney disease is diagnosed through blood tests; that's why you should have your kidney function checked via a blood test every six months. Normalizing blood pressure and blood sugar are the most effective ways of avoiding diabetic kidney disease. If you follow our diet recommendations for Diabetes, starting in Chapter Six you have an excellent chance at avoiding nephropathy.

• Sexual dysfunction
• Sexual problems in men

Diabetes commonly causes sexual problems in men and women. It is estimated that 50 percent of diabetic men suffer with erectile dysfunction. This is defined as an inability to have an erection firm enough for sexual intercourse. This may be an ongoing problem or an occasional problem. Erectile dysfunction in diabetics is caused by damage to the nerves that travel to the penis and/or damaged blood vessels within the penis. High blood pressure and high cholesterol also increase the risk of erectile dysfunction, and these conditions are usually present in diabetic men. Sometimes erection difficulties are the first warning sign of Type 2 Diabetes; therefore every man with this condition should have a blood test for Diabetes, among other investigations.

Diabetic men can also have problems with ejaculation. Retrograde ejaculation is a condition where all or part of a man's semen enters his bladder rather than going out through the penis during ejaculation. This occurs when internal muscles called sphincters don't function properly. The semen does not irritate the bladder; it leaves the body during urination. It causes the urine to appear cloudy. Apart from noticing cloudy urine, a man will also find that he releases very little semen during ejaculation. High blood sugar and the resulting nerve damage are responsible for causing retrograde ejaculation.

One in three males with Diabetes develops a testosterone deficiency, also known as hypogonadism. The symptoms of testosterone deficiency include erectile dysfunction, reduced sex drive, increased abdominal fat, reduced bone density and muscle tone, and mood changes, including depression. Testosterone deficiency is also a common feature of Syndrome X and obesity in men. It develops for a number of reasons. Diabetic men usually have excess fat around their abdominal area; fat cells here contain high levels of an enzyme called aromatase, which converts testosterone into oestrogen. Diabetic men who are overweight commonly suffer with sleep apnoea, a condition linked to snoring, where breathing stops many times throughout the night. Sleep apnoea is known to cause a fall in testosterone levels because the lack of quality sleep affects the brain's regulation of hormone levels.

Luckily the combination of weight loss, reduced blood sugar and reduced blood insulin helps to restore normal testosterone levels in most diabetic men.

• Sexual problems in women

Diabetic women are more likely to experience problems with vaginal lubrication. Damage to nerves that stimulate cells that line the vagina can lead to vaginal dryness, causing pain or discomfort during intercourse. Another common problem is reduced sexual response. It is estimated that at least 35 percent of diabetic women have a reduced or absent sexual response, meaning they lose sensitivity in the genital area, have a reduced ability to become aroused and a constant or occasional inability to reach orgasm. Women with Diabetes are much more likely to experience thrush (vaginal yeast infection) and bladder infections (cystitis). All of these factors combine to put a big dampener on a woman's libido. For more information about restoring libido in women see the book *Hormone Replacement the Real Truth.*

In both men and women symptoms of sexual dysfunction can also be a side effect of blood pressure medication or cholesterol lowering medication. As you can see, problems with libido and sexual function sometimes have nothing at all to do with hormones and more to do with the quality of your diet, which affects nerve function and circulation.

• Nerve damage (neuropathy)

Nerve disease related to Diabetes commonly produces tingling sensations, numbness and a type of burning pain called neuropathic pain. Initially there is a subtle loss of sensation in the hands and feet. Nerve damage to the extremities of the body is called peripheral neuropathy. This sometimes occurs in older people who are not diabetic but they have higher blood sugar than is ideal. Diabetes can also cause damage to nerves of the autonomic nervous system, meaning the nerves that control bodily functions such as stomach contractions, defecation, urination and other internal processes. Eventually symptoms such as constipation, diarrhea, impaired heart function and inability to empty the bladder may develop.

Approximately 60 percent of people with Diabetes eventually develop neuropathy. Nerve damage is responsible for many of the complications of Diabetes; it is the leading cause of lower limb amputations in diabetics. You are more likely to develop neuropathy if you have poor control over your blood sugar or you have sustained high blood sugar.

• Faster rate of aging

According to medical research published in the journal *The Lancet*, "having Diabetes is the clinical equivalent of aging 15 years". One consequence is that diabetics are at greatly increased risk of fatal strokes and heart attacks much earlier in life. High blood sugar and insulin levels in type 2 diabetics promote inflammation and free radical damage to the body. Free radical damage to proteins such as collagen and elastin makes you appear older.

High blood sugar has a lot of damaging effects in your body. Glucose is sticky, and when there are large amounts of glucose in your bloodstream it attaches itself to many of the body's proteins. This process is called glycosylation (or glycation) and it is very harmful. Glycosylation of proteins changes their structure in a way that makes the proteins cross-link with each other. The proteins that have been damaged by high amounts of glucose in the bloodstream are called Advanced Glycosylation End-products (AGEs).

This is a fitting name because glucose does make you age more quickly. Glycosylation of proteins harms them in a way similar to cooking protein; these damaged proteins cannot perform their functions properly, leading to various health problems. Glucose binds to hemoglobin in your red blood cells and reduces their ability to bind with oxygen, thus depleting your energy levels. When glucose binds to collagen it causes it to lose flexibility. This will make your skin age more quickly and it will impair the function of organs, joints and tissues that are supported by collagen.

High levels of glucose in the bloodstream create a lot of free radical damage, inflammation and tissue damage. The body tries to repair this damage with the use of antioxidants found in fruits, vegetables, herbs, spices and other foods. Diabetics use up antioxidants at a much faster rate than healthy people; therefore they have a much greater requirement for them in their diet. See Chapter Nine for more information about antioxidants for diabetics.

• Immune system dysfunction

High blood sugar encourages bacterial and fungal infections. Diabetics are more likely to develop infections and are at greater risk of complications from simple infections. They also take longer to recover from infections. Common sites of infection include the bladder, kidneys, feet, skin, gums and vagina. Sometimes a recurrent skin or vaginal yeast infection is the clue that leads to the diagnosis of Diabetes.

Diabetics are also more likely to have chronic, hidden infections in their body, such as in the gums, sinuses, lungs and various organs of the body. Elevated blood levels of C-reactive protein, a marker of inflammation in the body is common in diabetics and one explanation for this elevation is chronic infection. Chronic infections increase the risk of heart disease because of the damage to artery walls they can cause.

Slow wound healing is common in diabetics, partly because they have poor circulation, caused by damage to blood vessels. People with Diabetes are also often deficient in the nutrients required for healing, including vitamin C, zinc, selenium and vitamin A. High levels of free radical activity in diabetics uses up these nutrients at a faster rate.

Another consequence of immune dysfunction and poor circulation in diabetics is the development of foot ulcers. These can form chronic infections that are extremely difficult to treat.

• Cognitive problems and depression

Recent studies have shown that compared to healthy people of the same age and sex, diabetics are twice as likely to develop Alzheimer's disease. It is thought that the high blood sugar, combined with blood vessel damage contributes to dementia by impeding blood flow to the brain. In Alzheimer's patients, amyloid protein builds up in the brain, while the same protein is deposited in the pancreas of type 2 diabetics. Most people with Type 2 Diabetes have excessive blood levels of insulin; too much insulin causes excessive inflammation in the body, which also contributes to brain damage. Researchers from the Medical University of South Carolina studied 7148 healthy adults who were given a series of cognitive tests at the beginning of the study and followed up six years later. Results showed that the people with the highest blood level of insulin had significantly greater declines in delayed word recall and first letter word fluency.[12]

High blood glucose is also known to impair concentration and memory. It can make your thinking foggy and impair your ability to think quickly. For detailed information on how to protect your brain against Alzheimer's disease see the book *Alzheimer's: What you must know to protect your brain.*

Depression is thought to be twice as common in diabetics as the general population. Many different factors contribute to the development of depression, including emotions, biology and environmental factors. In diabetics, depression can be triggered by the restrictions and lifestyle adjustments that must be made, and also by the reduced quality of life Diabetes produces. It is also thought that the increased levels of inflammation in the body caused by high blood sugar influences the brain chemistry in a way that makes depression more likely to develop. Unfortunately depression makes people less motivated to eat well and exercise, resulting in poorer control of blood sugar and more complications of Diabetes.

• Foot problems

Diabetes can cause problems with the feet for two main reasons. One of these is nerve damage (neuropathy) to the nerves in your legs and feet. If the nerves here are damaged you will be less able to feel pain, heat and cold. You may develop a cut on your foot and not notice it for some time. The cut could become infected, and because diabetics have poor wound healing, it could become serious.

The second reason diabetics are more prone to foot problems is because of damage to blood vessels. Peripheral vascular disease means damage to small blood vessels away from the heart, such as in the feet and hands. Infections in the feet that are slow to heal place you at risk of developing ulcers or even gangrene, which is death of tissue due to a lack of blood. Unfortunately this sometimes leads to the need for amputation. Diabetics are more prone to fungal infections of the feet (athlete's foot) and persistent fungal nail infections. It is vital to check your feet every day and alert your doctor to any problems straight away.

• Tooth and gum problems

People with Diabetes are more susceptible to developing infections of the gums and bones that hold the teeth in place. High blood sugar can cause a dry mouth and the lack of saliva can increase the risk of plaque and bacterial buildup. This means diabetics are more prone to tooth decay, painful and bleeding gums, gum infections and bad breath. Therefore the six monthly visit to the dentist is especially important for diabetics.

• Osteoporosis

Women who have had Type 2 Diabetes for 12 years or more are three times more likely to experience a hip fracture than non-diabetic women.

• Enlarged prostate

Research has shown that diabetic men are more than twice as likely to experience BPH (benign prostatic hypertrophy) than non-diabetic men. The risk of BPH increases with obesity and elevated blood sugar.

5. Medication used in the treatment of Type 2 Diabetes

People with type 1 Diabetes must inject insulin several times a day. There are different forms of insulin; they are categorized by how quickly they begin acting, and how long their action lasts. Insulin is also used in type 2 diabetics whose Diabetes has progressed to an advanced stage and in women with gestational Diabetes if diet changes don't bring blood sugar down.

People with Type 2 Diabetes may be either diet controlled, meaning they make changes to their diet and perform regular exercise to control their Diabetes, or they take tablets. There are several categories of oral Diabetes tablets. These drugs may be used alone or in combination:

Oral Diabetes medication

• **Sulfonylureas:** Some examples of the first generation sulfonylurea drugs include tolazamide, acetohexamide, gliclazide (*Diamicron, Glyade*) and glipizide (*Glucotrol, Melizide, Minidiab*). They are not used much today because they are less potent and shorter acting than the newer sulfonylureas, which include glimepiride (*Amaryl*) and glyburide (*Diabeta, Glynase, Micronase, Daonil*).

How they work: Sulfonylureas lower blood sugar by stimulating the pancreas to release more insulin. They do this by making insulin secreting cells in the pancreas more sensitive to glucose. Sulfonylureas only work if there are some functional pancreatic cells left that are capable of producing insulin. They can reduce HbA$_{1c}$ by approximately 1 to 2 percent. Sulfonylureas are usually used in combination with another drug.

Potential problems: These drugs lose their effectiveness over time. Because they stimulate greater insulin release by the pancreas, this class of drugs promotes weight gain and will make losing weight harder. Inability to lose weight is something most diabetics already struggle with, therefore over the long term sulfonylureas may lead to a worsening of Diabetes.

The main side effect of sulfonylureas is Hypoglycemia (low blood sugar). Some people experience allergic skin reactions to the drugs, or indigestion, nausea, vomiting, headache or fatigue. In a minority of people these drugs can cause liver damage. Sulfonylureas should NOT be used in the following circumstances:

- Pregnancy

- Allergy to sulfa drugs

- During long term corticosteroid treatment

- During injury, surgery or infection

- **Biguanides:** The only drug in this category is metformin; some brand names include *Glucophage, Diaformin, Diabex and Glucomet.*

How they work: These drugs inhibit the liver from releasing stored glucose. They also improve the ability of insulin to transport sugar into cells, especially muscle cells. Therefore they make your body more sensitive to insulin. Biguanides can lower blood glucose by 13 to 35 percent and HbA1c by 1.5 to 2 percent.

A positive side effect of metformin is that it promotes weight loss. It also helps to reduce triglycerides and LDL "bad" cholesterol while increasing HDL "good" cholesterol.

Potential problems: The following side effects are quite common: diarrhea, abdominal bloating, flatulence, nausea and vomiting. Thankfully these symptoms tend to lessen with time. Unfortunately metformin can cause you to become deficient in vitamin B12. You should have a blood test for this vitamin once a year if you take metformin. This drug can cause a metallic taste in the mouth.

Metformin should not be used in people with kidney damage, heart failure and must be used with caution in the elderly. This is because it may produce a rare but serious side effect called lactic acidosis. This is where lactic acid builds up in the body and makes the bloodstream too acidic.

- **Thiazolidinediones:** Examples of this class of drugs include pioglitazone (*Actos)* and rosiglitazone *(Avandia).*

How they work: These drugs reduce the amount of glucose released by the liver and increase the sensitivity of fat and muscle cells to insulin. It may take a few weeks for these drugs to start working and produce their blood sugar lowering effect. They can reduce HbA_{1c} by 1 to 2 percent. Of all the oral Type 2 Diabetes drugs, these are the most effective at restoring fertility in women with polycystic ovarian syndrome.

Potential problems: The first drug in this category (troglitazone, brand name *Rezulin*) was taken off the market because it caused widespread deaths due to liver failure. *Actos* and *Avandia* have not been shown to cause serious liver disease, but it is essential to have a liver function test every two months in the first year you take one of these drugs, and then annually after that.

Thiazolidinediones promote weight gain and raise triglycerides and LDL "bad" cholesterol in most people. They also commonly produce mild to moderate fluid retention. They should be used with caution in people with heart failure because of their tendency to increase fluid retention. These drugs cause headaches in some people and may make you more susceptible to respiratory infections.

A new study conducted in New Zealand has shown that people taking Avandia are at greater risk of bone fractures because the drug decreases bone formation. A study of 50 postmenopausal women showed that those taking Avandia had a 1.9 percent drop in total hip bone density after only 14 weeks of treatment. The women taking a placebo had a reduction of 0.2 percent.[13] Diabetics are already more prone to osteoporosis, therefore this new study is cause for concern. Recent research has shown these drugs increase the risk of heart attacks and heart failure.

- **Alpha-glucosidase inhibitors:** Acarbose *(Precose, Glucobay)* is the name of the drug in this category.

How it works: This drug blocks the action of enzymes that digest carbohydrates, thereby slowing the digestion of carbohydrate in the small intestine. This means sugar is absorbed into the bloodstream much more slowly. Acarbose can lower HbA_{1c} by 0.5 to 1 percent.

Potential problems: This drug can cause diarrhea, flatulence, abdominal cramps and nausea.

• **Meglitinides:** Repaglinide *(Prandin, NovoNorm)* is the name of the drug in this category.

How it works: This drug stimulates the pancreas to release a surge of insulin immediately after you eat. This drug only stimulates the pancreas to release more insulin if blood sugar is high, whereas sulfonylureas cause insulin to be released irrespective of blood sugar levels. Therefore repaglinide is a lot less likely to cause Hypoglycemia.

Potential problems: Repaglinide can cause an upset stomach, diarrhea, constipation, headaches and chest pains.

6. Reversing Type 2 Diabetes through diet

In this section we will discuss the three major food groups: protein, fat and carbohydrate, their significance in your diet and their effects on Diabetes. Traditionally diabetics are told to base their diet on carbohydrate rich foods, but for the reasons described in the following pages, we strongly disagree with this recommendation.

All about protein

Protein is made up of building blocks called amino acids. There are eight essential amino acids that your body requires. We call them essential because your body cannot manufacture them, therefore must obtain them through your diet. Through digestion, enzymes break dietary protein into amino acids in the small intestine. Once inside your body, these amino acids can be reassembled into muscles, organs, nerves, enzymes, neurotransmitters and hormones. Protein can also be converted into glucose in your body but this is a slow and inefficient process.

Protein is found in many foods; the richest source is animal foods such as red meat, eggs, seafood, poultry and dairy products; apart from dairy products, these foods contain virtually no carbohydrate. Protein is found in smaller quantities in plant foods such as legumes (beans, lentils), nuts, seeds and grains; these foods also contain varying quantities of carbohydrate and fat.

A protein food is considered a **complete protein** if it contains all eight essential amino acids; this is also called **first class protein**.

Animal foods contain first class proteins and plant foods do not. Examples of first class proteins include:

- Red meat
- Poultry
- Seafood
- Eggs
- Whey protein powder

- Cheese and yogurt contain some protein but are best combined with one of the foods above to achieve a complete protein.

Vegetarians and vegans can combine three of the following at the same meal to achieve complete protein: a nut, a seed, a legume and a grain. Since grains are the richest source of carbohydrate, we recommend they be completely avoided while trying to reverse Type 2 Diabetes. If you are a vegetarian or a vegan you can combine a nut with a seed with a legume, however a meal like this is much higher in carbohydrate than a meal consisting of fish and salad for instance, therefore weight loss and blood sugar lowering will be much slower. Our meal plan in Chapter Eleven does not contain any recipes suitable for vegetarians for this reason; however there are suitable recipes in Chapter Twelve.

The body cannot convert carbohydrate or fat into protein.

Eating protein does not cause a significant rise in blood sugar or insulin.

Protein is the most important nutrient in your diet to control your Diabetes and lose weight.

Protein will help you lose weight

Most people with Type 2 Diabetes are overweight and find it incredibly difficult to lose weight. Losing weight is an essential part of reversing Type 2 Diabetes because it will improve your body's sensitivity to insulin and bring your blood sugar down. Many studies have shown that diets higher in protein (comprising 25 to 35 percent of total energy intake) result in weight loss. Protein helps you lose weight in several ways:

- Eating protein makes you feel full. Protein has a two to three times greater satiety value than carbohydrate or fat, so people tend to eat less when they eat more protein. Out of fat, carbohydrate and protein. Protein causes the greatest release of a hormone secreted by the gut called PYY. This hormone reduces hunger and also improves your body's sensitivity to the hormone leptin, which reduces appetite and regulates your body fat stores.

• Protein has a greater thermic effect than fat or carbohydrate, meaning it requires more energy to be digested than the other nutrients. Research has shown that after a meal, energy expenditure by your body increases zero to three percent for the metabolism of fat, five to ten percent for carbohydrate and a whopping 20 to 30 percent for protein![14] The greatest increase in thermogenesis occurs after eating animal derived protein, such as fish, eggs, chicken or meat, rather than soy or other plant protein.[15]

• Protein does not cause a significant rise in blood sugar or insulin levels, therefore eating more protein can help to reduce insulin resistance. Eating protein at each meal helps to keep your blood sugar level stable and this reduces the tendency to develop Hypoglycemia or sugar/carbohydrate cravings.

• In addition to weight loss, higher protein diets help to improve cholesterol levels and reduce blood triglyceride levels.

Therefore, eating protein makes you feel full faster, causing you to eat less, while expending more energy during digestion and metabolism! All helping you to lose weight.

Studies have shown that higher protein diets help diabetics lose weight

A recent study published in the *International Journal of Obesity* placed 93 overweight insulin resistant (meaning they have Syndrome X) women on one of three diets: high protein, high fat or high carbohydrate. The study aimed to determine which dietary regime offered best results in terms of weight loss, body composition and blood fat levels. The trial ran for 12 months and the women were interviewed and assessed at the half way point and again at the end.

The results showed that 93 percent of the women on the high protein diet stuck with the diet for a whole year, whereas the rate was 75 percent for the high fat and high carbohydrate group. Overall, the study found that women on the high protein diet experienced clinically significant improvements in waist circumference, body fat levels, fasting triglyceride and insulin levels and weight loss, above both the high fat and high carbohydrate groups.

Significantly, these benefits remained for the 12 month duration of the diet, whereas women in the other groups noticed weight loss and other improvements in the first six months, but by the 12 month period the benefits had started to reverse. Women in the high carbohydrate group lost the least amount of weight and those on the high fat diet regressed so rapidly that any initial benefits were quickly lost.[16]

Another study published in the journal Diabetes Care showed the effectiveness of higher protein diets for diabetics. The study is titled *"A hypocaloric high-protein diet as primary therapy for adults with obesity-related Diabetes: effective long-term use in a community hospital"*.[17] Researchers placed 36 obese type 2 diabetic patients who were on insulin therapy on a higher protein diet consisting of 1.7 to 2.0 grams of protein per day per kilo of body weight. This is significantly more protein than conventional recommendations; according to the World Health Organization we only need 0.6 grams of protein per day per kilo of body weight.

This study lasted 41 weeks and at the end, eight patients lost weight and achieved normal blood sugar levels. Twenty patients lost some weight then plateaued but continued to have normal blood sugar. Only eight patients needed to remain on insulin to control their blood sugar. The study concluded with the following statement:

This hypocaloric high-protein diet thus appears to be a generally successful means of weaning obese diabetic adult patients from insulin. This can be done rapidly, safely and permanently in the community. Such diet therapy appears to require minimal laboratory and hospital resources that are available to all health care providers.

If you are on insulin therapy please speak to your doctor before making any dietary changes. Do not attempt to discontinue insulin therapy without your doctor's approval.

Protein does not cause kidney disease

Kidney disease (nephropathy) is a common long term complication of Diabetes. Some people with severe kidney disease must restrict their protein intake because one of the kidneys' jobs is to remove the waste products of protein digestion from your blood. However, diabetics who do not have kidney disease are often cautioned on eating protein in the mistaken belief that it may hasten the development of diabetic nephropathy.

People are commonly told that eating too much protein will "over work" or "strain" their kidneys. This is not correct. Eating protein does not cause kidney disease in non-diabetics and diabetics who maintain near-normal blood sugar and blood pressure do not get kidney disease. Diabetic nephropathy is caused by high blood sugar and high blood pressure, not by eating protein. The higher your HbA_{1c}, the more likely you are to develop diabetic nephropathy.[18]

How much protein do you need?

Diabetics must consume first class protein at every meal. This means a type of protein that contains all eight essential amino acids. Suitable forms of protein include seafood, poultry, eggs, whey protein powder and red meat. These types of protein are beneficial for diabetics because they contain virtually no carbohydrate and they can be low in fat, depending on the specific types chosen.

It is also possible to obtain first class protein by combining three of the following at the same meal: legume, nut, seed or grain. However, because these foods are fairly high in carbohydrate, they are not recommended to form the basis of your meals while trying to bring down your blood sugar. You must avoid all grains while trying to reverse Type 2 Diabetes, but can eat small amounts of legumes, nuts and seeds. You will find that these foods are not featured in the main meals of our eating plan in Chapter Eleven.

All about Fat

Fats are also known as lipids and they are composed of fatty acids. Fatty acids are chains of carbon atoms with hydrogen atoms filling up available bonds. The fat you eat in your diet is broken down into fatty acids by bile and digestive enzymes. Most of the fats in our body are triglycerides, which are three fatty acids attached to one glycerol molecule. Fatty acids can be classified as saturated, monounsaturated and polyunsaturated.

All types of fat have vital roles in our body and we need small to moderate amounts of all of them for good health. Some of the benefits of fat include:

- They provide structure and integrity to your cell membranes.

- They increase the satiety of a meal, helping to make you feel full so that you are less likely to crave sugar and high carbohydrate foods.

- They enhance the function of your immune system.

- They help you absorb the fat soluble vitamins A, D, E and K, as well as transport them around your body.

- Fat provides your body with insulation and cushions your organs.

Saturated fats are usually solid at room temperature; they are commonly found in animal foods such as butter, full fat dairy products and tropical oils like coconut oil and palm oil. Saturated fats are highly stable, meaning they do not readily become rancid, or go off. They tolerate heat well and do not easily become oxidized. This makes them quite suitable for cooking.

Monounsaturated fats are usually liquid at room temperature and become solid when refrigerated. They are fairly stable and do not become rancid or oxidized easily; this means they can be used in cooking. The most common monounsaturated fat in most people's diet is oleic acid, which is found in great quantities in olive oil. Other foods high in monounsaturated fat include macadamia nuts, avocados and peanuts.

Polyunsaturated fats are liquid at room temperature and remain liquid even when refrigerated. There are two types of polyunsaturated fats: omega 6 fats and omega 3 fats. Most people get plenty of omega 6 fats in their diet; in fact they are likely to consume too much of this type of fat, which can lead to health problems. Omega 6 fats are abundant in common vegetable oils such as sunflower, safflower, sesame and corn oil. Margarine and most kinds of cooking oils are very high in omega 6 fats. The problem with these fats is they are highly unstable and reactive, meaning they easily react with oxygen, light, water and various molecules in the body. Once this happens the fats act like free radicals in your body and promote inflammation. In this way, a high intake of omega 6 fats can promote the development of heart disease, cancer and Diabetes.

A very beneficial type of polyunsaturated fat is called omega 3 fat. Alpha-linolenic acid (ALA) is an omega 3 fat found in flaxseeds, walnuts, pecans and a few vegetables (in tiny quantities). Our body converts ALA into two types of omega 3 fatty acids called eicosapentaenoic acid (EPA) and docosahexaenoic acid (DHA); however this process is quite inefficient. A more reliable way to obtain beneficial EPA and DHA is through eating oily fish such as salmon, sardines, herrings, anchovies and mackerel.

Both omega 6 and omega 3 fatty acids are called essential fatty acids; meaning we must obtain them in our diet because our body cannot manufacture them.

Your body can manufacture other types of fats, depending on what is needed at the time. In other instances, your body makes large amounts of saturated fat out of sugar and high carbohydrate foods like bread, pasta and potatoes that you eat but don't burn off as energy.

Omega 3 fatty acids are extremely beneficial for diabetics; they have the following benefits in your body:

- They lower blood triglyceride levels.
- They lower blood pressure.
- They make your platelets less sticky, therefore reducing the risk of blood clots forming, which can lead to heart attacks and strokes.
- They reduce the risk of cardiac arrhythmias (disturbances in the heart's rhythm that can lead to a heart attack).
- They increase your metabolic rate and help you burn fat more efficiently.
- They decrease the rate of plaque accumulation in the arteries.
- They have an anti inflammatory effect in your body.

- They have mood enhancing effects and help to prevent depression.
- They help to stabilise arterial plaques, making them less likely to rupture and lead to a heart attack.
- They increase blood levels of HDL "good" cholesterol.
- They can help to break up blood clots already present in the body.

Trans Fatty Acids

These fats should be strictly avoided by everyone, especially diabetics. Trans fatty acids are artificial, man made fats. They are derived from vegetable oils, and manufactured by forcing hydrogen atoms into their fatty acid chain. They then become **hydrogenated** or **partially hydrogenated vegetable oil**. This makes the fat more solid at room temperature. Trans fats are found in many processed baked goods such as chips/crisps, cookies, cakes and pastries. They are popular with food manufacturers because they are cheap and have a long shelf life. To determine if a food contains trans fatty acids look for the words "partially hydrogenated vegetable oil", "hydrogenated vegetable oil" or "vegetable fat" on the label and avoid it.

Fats largely make up our cell membranes. If we eat a lot of trans fatty acids we develop weakened cell membranes, which affects the cells' ability to communicate with various substances. Trans fats are said to promote Syndrome X and Diabetes because they impair the communication between insulin and the cell membrane; hence higher amounts of insulin need to be secreted after a meal.

Trans fats clog the liver and promote the development of fatty liver disease; they can also raise LDL "bad" cholesterol and lower HDL "good" cholesterol.

Should you follow a low fat diet?

For many years diabetics have been told they must restrict their fat intake for two main reasons: to lose weight and to reduce their risk of heart disease. We don't believe fat is responsible for either of these conditions and will elaborate on why.

Myth Number 1:
Eating fat makes you fat

The belief that eating fat makes you fat is too simplistic and not entirely accurate. It is true that fat is high in calories and if you eat a great deal of it you will gain weight. But type 2 diabetics are overweight because they are insulin resistant, meaning they have high levels of insulin in their body which the body is no longer responding to. Insulin promotes your body to store fat and inhibits your body from burning fat.

Eating fat does not promote a rise in blood sugar or insulin levels. However, eating high carbohydrate food, like a bowl of pasta will cause a rise in your blood sugar level, followed by a rise in your insulin level. The blood sugar that is not burnt off as energy or converted into glycogen is converted into body fat and stored, particularly over the abdominal area, where most diabetics carry excess weight. If a farmer wants to fatten his cows or pigs he doesn't feed them butter, eggs and red meat; he feeds them grain. We are the same; if you want to fatten yourself up eat lots of bread, pasta, breakfast cereals, potatoes and rice. If you eat a lot of these foods your insulin level will remain high, which inhibits your body from burning fat. You don't have to eat any fat to be overweight.

Myth Number 2:
Eating fat raises your risk of heart disease

A high intake of dietary fat is typically blamed for high cholesterol and triglyceride levels but this is not the case. You don't need to eat any fat at all to have a high cholesterol level. Approximately 80 percent of the cholesterol in your body is made in your liver and the rest comes from your diet. You can be a vegetarian or vegan and still have high cholesterol levels.

The enzyme in your liver that is responsible for cholesterol production is stimulated by insulin; so insulin instructs your liver to manufacture greater amounts of cholesterol and triglycerides. It produces them mainly from starch and carbohydrate in your diet, or any calories in excess of your needs. Any sugar and carbohydrate that your body does not burn off for energy can be turned into cholesterol and triglycerides in your liver. The fact that most type 2 diabetics have a fatty liver means their liver will be making large quantities of LDL "bad" cholesterol and triglycerides. The only fat that raises LDL "bad" cholesterol and lowers HDL "good" cholesterol is trans fatty acids.

If eating fat doesn't cause heart disease, what does? Excessive levels of inflammation in the body cause damage to the inner lining of blood vessels, promoting the development of fatty plaques. A number of factors promote inflammation, including:

- Being overweight
- Diabetes
- Stress
- Cigarette smoking
- A lack of antioxidants in the diet
- Infections
- Immune system disorders, such as autoimmune disease

Cholesterol is involved in the process of heart disease but it is not the initiating factor. When the cholesterol that is in your body becomes oxidized (via free radical damage) it adheres to your artery walls much more readily. This reinforces the need for antioxidants in your diet. For detailed information on the role of inflammation in heart disease please see our book *Cholesterol the Real Truth*.

Eating sugar is known to raise the risk of heart disease. A study published in the journal The Lancet found that men who had a heart attack ate almost twice the amount of sugar as men who haven't had a heart attack. In people with coronary heart disease, the degree of atherosclerosis is proportional to the amount of refined sugar consumed.[19]

Healthy fats for diabetics

Omega 3 fats in oily fish

Olive oil

Macadamia nut oil

Ground flaxseeds

Raw nuts and seeds

Avocados

Eggs

Unhealthy fats for diabetics

Trans fatty acids found in some vegetable oil and margarine.

Polyunsaturated vegetable oil

All about Carbohydrate

Carbohydrates are basically different forms of sugar, linked together in chains. All plant foods including grains, starches, fiber, vegetables and fruits, nuts and seeds and legumes contain carbohydrate. Grains are the richest source of carbohydrate. Dairy products contain small amounts of the carbohydrate lactose.

In the past, carbohydrates were divided up into two main groups: simple carbohydrates and complex carbohydrates. Simple carbohydrates are things like table sugar (sucrose), fruit sugar (fructose), glucose and dextrose. Simple carbohydrates were always considered to be bad for your health if eaten in large quantities. Complex carbohydrates are made of three or more linked sugars, they include things like bread, potatoes and pasta; they _were_ always considered to be good for your health.

In reality, all carbohydrates are digested into sugar (glucose); it doesn't matter if the carbohydrates are simple, complex, high or low fiber, high glycemic or low glycemic; in the end all carbohydrates are broken down into glucose and raise your blood sugar level.

You may remember that there are essential fatty acids (omega 3 and 6), which you must obtain in your diet and essential amino acids (eight amino acids) but there are no essential carbohydrates. You do not need to eat grains and cereals to obtain enough carbohydrate in your diet. All plant food (including vegetables) contains adequate carbohydrate for healthy body function.

What about glycemic index (GI)?

The glycemic index is a more useful tool than knowing whether a carbohydrate is simple or complex. It measures how fast your blood sugar rises after consuming a particular food. Pure glucose is given a rating of 100 and all other foods are measured against it. Foods with a high glycemic index are rapidly digested and cause a rapid rise in your blood sugar level and insulin level; eating them is also more likely to lead to an unstable blood sugar level and weight gain. Foods with a low glycemic index are slowly digested and produce a much slower rise in blood sugar. They cause only a moderate rise in blood sugar and insulin levels and help with weight loss.

- A food is considered to have a high GI if it is greater than 70.

- A food is considered to have a moderate GI if it is between 56 and 70.

- A food is considered to have a low GI if it is less than 55.

Diabetics and people with Syndrome X should consume foods with a low glycemic index. Foods that do not contain any carbohydrate at all, for example eggs, red meat and fish have a glycemic index of zero. No carbs means no glycemic index. Most vegetables, apart from starchy vegetables like potato and parsnip have an extremely low GI.

Glycemic Load

A more useful measure than glycemic index is glycemic load. It takes into account the quantity of carbohydrate in a serving of food. The glycemic index only tells you how rapidly a carbohydrate food turns into blood sugar; it doesn't tell you how much carbohydrate is present in that food. For example, a food like watermelon has a GI of 72, which is high, but there is so little carbohydrate present in a typical serve of watermelon that it's really not significant. In comparison, a cup of white rice has a GI of 72 also, but it contains far more carbohydrate, therefore has a much more significant effect on your blood sugar, insulin level and weight.

How to measure the glycemic load (GL)

To determine the glycemic load of a food, divide the glycemic index of a food by 100 and multiply that by the carbohydrate content (in grams) of a serving of food.

For example, a medium Bartlett pear weighing 120 grams contains 11.3 grams of carbohydrate and has a GI of 41. To determine its glycemic load we use the following formula:

- 41 divided by 100 = 0.41

- 0.41 x 11.3 = 4.63

Therefore the GL of a medium Bartlett pear is 4.63, which is low.

- A Glycemic Load of 20 or more is considered high

- A Glycemic Load of 11 to 19 is medium

- A Glycemic Load of 10 or less is low

Eating foods with a high glycemic load raises blood sugar and triglycerides and increases the risk of Diabetes and heart disease.

Glycemic index and glycemic load are useful tools to determine the impact of foods on your blood sugar and insulin levels, however it is not essential to use them if you follow our Diabetes meal plan in Chapter Eleven.

To reverse Type 2 Diabetes and lose weight you must reduce the total carbohydrate content of your diet. By following our meal plan you will automatically be on a low glycemic index and low glycemic load diet.

Is sugar any worse than bread and potatoes?

Sugar has always been thought of as a very unhealthy food for diabetics and that's true. The interesting thing is that sucrose, commonly known as table sugar only has a moderate glycemic index, so it certainly isn't a rapidly absorbed carbohydrate. There are many other commonly eaten foods that have a much higher glycemic index and are much worse for diabetics, these include: potatoes, most bread, most rice, some pasta and the great majority of breakfast cereals.

This just reinforces the fact that **all carbohydrates are digested into sugar** in the end and they should be severely restricted in the diets of type 2 diabetics. If you regularly consume foods high in carbohydrate (like all diabetics are told to do), much of the glucose you don't use immediately will be converted into body fat. Your body will never get the opportunity to burn its own fat stores and you will remain overweight. If plenty of glucose is always circulating around in your bloodstream why would your body go through the harder process of breaking down your fat stores for energy?

Studies show that diabetics are healthier on a low carbohydrate diet

Several studies have been conducted proving the fact that low carbohydrate diets are appropriate for type 2 diabetics. Even the Stanford University School of Medicine says that low fat diets aggravate insulin resistance and diabetics should be consuming less carbohydrate.

A review of low carbohydrate diets in the management of Type 2 Diabetes was published in the medical journal called *Nutrition and Metabolism* and titled *The case for low carbohydrate diets in Diabetes management*. After reviewing many studies utilizing low carbohydrate diets the researchers came to the following conclusions:

"A high carbohydrate diet raises postprandial (post meal) plasma glucose and insulin secretion, thereby increasing risk of cardiovascular disease, hypertension, dyslipidaemia (elevated cholesterol and triglycerides), obesity and Diabetes. Moreover, the current epidemic of Diabetes and obesity has been, over the past three decades, accompanied by a significant decrease in fat consumption and an increase in carbohydrate consumption". The review also stated *"Furthermore, the ability of low carbohydrate diets to reduce triglycerides and to increase HDL is of particular importance."*[20]

Another study published in the same journal is titled *A low carbohydrate diet may prevent end stage renal failure in Type 2 Diabetes*. This study explains how following a low carbohydrate diet helps with weight loss and blood sugar control, thereby reducing the risk of kidney disease. The study made the following interesting comments:

"Metabolic control in such patients (type 2 diabetics) is, however, difficult because the recommended low fat diet with its high content of carbohydrates usually leads to a vicious cycle: Hyperglycemia (high blood sugar) caused by the high carbohydrate diet necessitates the use of insulin; efforts to normalize the blood glucose with insulin injections leads to increase of appetite and body weight; the rise of body weight exposes the patient to the risk of obesity-associated renal failure".[21]

This study looked at advanced Type 2 Diabetes, whereby the patient needs to be on insulin therapy. The use of insulin further increases the risk of kidney damage because it promotes weight gain.

Artificial sweeteners

In order for people to continue enjoying sweet tasting foods and beverages while avoiding sugar, artificially sweetened products have flourished. Sugar free and low carb foods are a booming industry, with alternatives for most sugary snacks now readily available.

Avoiding sugar is important for diabetics, but make sure the sugar substitutes you consume aren't even more harmful.

The following artificial sweeteners should be avoided:

• **Aspartame:** The main brands are NutraSweet and Equal. Aspartame is made of phenylalanine, aspartic acid and methanol (a kind of alcohol). In the body, methanol breaks down into formaldehyde (a cancer causing substance); formic acid (an acid found in the venom of bees and ants); and diketopiperazine (shown to cause brain tumors in animals). **Aspartame can be identified on food labels by the food additive number 951.**

• **Sucralose**: This is marketed as Splenda. Sucralose is made from sugar, by chlorinating sucrose. Three chlorine atoms are substituted for three hydroxyl groups in the sugar molecule. Sucralose is a relatively new sweetener, being approved in 1991 in Canada, and 1998 in the USA. It was approved for use in Australia by the National Food Authority in October 1993. Pre-approval research in the USA showed that sucralose caused the thymus gland of rats to shrink by up to 40 percent when taken in large doses. The thymus gland is an organ in the chest responsible for the development of the immune system. **Sucralose can be identified by the number 955.**

• **Acesulfame-K**: This is a derivative of acetoacetic acid and was approved by the FDA in 1998. The risks of long term damage from consumption of this sweetener are not known. **Acesulfame-K is listed as food additive 950.**

• **Saccharin**: This sweetener was discovered in 1879 and is approximately 300 times sweeter than sugar. Studies have shown that large doses may cause cancer in laboratory animals. Risks to humans are not known. **Saccharin is additive number 954.**

• **Cyclamate**: is 30 times sweeter than sucrose and is heat-stable. It has been used widely in diet foods and beverages since its discovery in 1937. Cyclamate has been approved for use in more than 80 countries and is often used together with other sweeteners. **Cyclamate can be identified as 952.**

• **Alitame**: This sweetener is approximately 2, 000 times sweeter than sucrose and is approved in Australia, Europe and China. It is composed of the two amino acids alanine and aspartic acid. **You can identify it by the number 956.**

Healthy Sweeteners for Diabetics

The following sweeteners are all naturally derived from plants and are recommended for diabetics:

• **Stevia:** This is an herbal sweetener that has been used for centuries in South America and for 30 years in Japan. Steviosides are the molecules that make stevia taste sweet, and they were first identified in 1931. Stevia contains no calories and has no effect on blood sugar levels; hence it is a great alternative for those watching their weight and blood sugar. You can find stevia in tablet, powder or liquid form; it can be used conveniently in tea, coffee or cooking. If you would like more information about stevia and how to use it, please call our Health Advisory line in the USA on 623 334 3232 or in Australia on 02 4655 8855.

• **Xylitol, Maltitol, Mannitol, Lactitol, Sorbitol**: These are classed as sugar alcohols, or polyols. Sugar alcohols are lower in calories than sucrose, and do not have as dramatic effect on blood sugar or insulin levels. These sweeteners are becoming increasingly common in sugar free foods, and some offer benefits against tooth decay. If consumed in large quantities, these sweeteners may cause digestive distress, such as abdominal bloating, cramps, flatulence or diarrhea.

• **Fructose:** This is the most abundant sugar in fruits. It has a low glycemic index of only 20. Fructose eaten in large quantities can promote the development of fatty liver and Syndrome X. It is acceptable to use in small quantities only.

• **Thaumatin**: This is a protein derived from the katemfe fruit of west Africa. It is mostly found in brewed soda pops and is represented by the number 957. It is not commonly used in Australia.

• **Agave syrup/nectar**: This is a natural sweetener derived from the Agave plant which is native to Mexico and parts of America. Agave does contain calories; is approximately 25 percent sweeter than sugar and has a lower glycemic index than sugar. It is available from health food stores. It is fairly high in fructose, therefore please use it sparingly or not at all.

• Lifestyle Changes are More Effective than Drugs

People with Syndrome X who are overweight and don't exercise are at high risk of developing Type 2 Diabetes. Making diet changes and exercising regularly are better at preventing Type 2 Diabetes than drugs.

A study published in the *New England Journal of Medicine* set out to prove this theory. More than 3,200 non-diabetic men and women with an average age of 51 were studied. All of them had above normal blood glucose levels and their average body mass index was 34 (obese category). The participants were divided into three groups; one third were given a placebo, another third were given 850mg of the Diabetes drug metformin twice daily and one third were put on a lifestyle change program where they engaged in 150 minutes of exercise each week and had help to lose at least seven percent of their body weight.

The study lasted almost three years. At the end it was clear that the group on the lifestyle change program experienced the greatest reduction in their risk of Diabetes. This group had a 58 percent lower risk of developing Type 2 Diabetes than the placebo group. The people taking metformin cut their Diabetes risk by 31 percent. Clearly Type 2 Diabetes is caused by poor lifestyle choices; therefore the cure for this disease is making improvements in diet and exercise choices.[22]

Specific beneficial foods for diabetics

Some foods have specific benefits for diabetics, they include:

• Nuts

Many people are afraid of eating nuts because they are high in fat. That is true but the fats they contain are extremely beneficial and are unlikely to cause weight gain when part of a healthy diet. Several studies have shown that people who eat nuts regularly are less likely to be overweight than people who don't eat them and less likely to suffer heart disease.

A recent study showed women who regularly consume nuts are much less likely to develop Type 2 Diabetes irrespective of their risk factors for the disease, such as family history, physical activity and other dietary factors. The interesting part is that nuts even protected obese women from developing Type 2 Diabetes.[23]

Nuts are high in beneficial monounsaturated and polyunsaturated fatty acids, which improve cell membrane health and insulin sensitivity. They are also an excellent source of fiber and magnesium, are low in carbohydrate and have a low glycemic index. All of these factors make nuts extremely beneficial for diabetics.

Research done on almonds has shown they reduce post-meal glucose levels and reduce the formation of advanced glycosylation end products; meaning they reduce damage done to proteins in the body by glucose.[24]

This is very significant for diabetics because glucose levels are highest after a meal and this is the time glucose does most of its harm to the body. The formation of advanced glycosylation end products is responsible for many of the long term health complications of Diabetes.

Nuts and seeds should be consumed in their natural state, unroasted and preferably unsalted. Because they are high in calories it is best to limit your consumption of nuts and seeds to one handful a day.

• Cherries

Researchers from Michigan State University have found that naturally occurring chemicals in cherries help to fight Diabetes. Laboratory tests done on animal pancreatic cells found that compounds called anthocyanins increased insulin production by 50 percent and therefore helped to lower blood sugar.[25] Anthocyanins are also powerful antioxidants and they give cherries their vibrant color. They have a range of other benefits, including protection against heart disease and cancer.

If you are a diabetic, including some cherries in your diet can help you achieve better blood sugar control. Please remember that all fruit is fairly high in carbohydrate and should be limited to two serving sizes per day. A serving size could be one orange or approximately 12 cherries.

• Coffee

This is the news you've been waiting to hear; coffee is good for you! Well at least it may reduce your chances of developing Type 2 Diabetes. The news isn't that positive if you already have Diabetes.

A study conducted by researchers at the Harvard School of Public Health and Brigham and Women's Hospital tracked more than 125,000 people who were free of Diabetes, cardiovascular disease and cancer at the beginning of the study. 41,934 men were assessed between 1986 and 1998 and 84,276 women were monitored between 1980 and 1998. The participants were given food frequency questionnaires to determine their intake of regular and decaffeinated coffee over that time.

During the study there were 1,333 cases of newly diagnosed Type 2 Diabetes in men and 4,085 cases in women. Researchers were startled to find that men who drank more than six cups of caffeinated coffee per day reduced their risk of Type 2 Diabetes by 50 percent, compared to men who didn't drink coffee. When it came to women, those who drank the same amount of coffee reduced their risk by almost 30 percent. These findings could not be explained by lifestyle factors such as smoking, obesity or exercise. Decaffeinated coffee offered some benefits against Diabetes, but they were much weaker.[26]

Coffee contains large amounts of the antioxidant chlorogenic acid (which is partly responsible for the flavour of coffee), plus magnesium. Both of these substances improve insulin sensitivity and reduce the risk of Type 2 Diabetes.

However, coffee does raise blood sugar in the short term and if you are already a diabetic, drinking coffee will make it harder to control your blood sugar and lose weight. There are much healthier ways to reduce your risk of Type 2 Diabetes than drinking copious amounts of coffee. Six cups of coffee a day promotes the loss of calcium from your bones into your urine; it aggravates high blood pressure, anxiety and insomnia and raises the risk of miscarriage. Coffee is also a heavily sprayed crop and exposes you to many pesticides unless it is organic. If you drink coffee it is best to limit it to two cups per day.

7. Conventional dietary recommendations for diabetics and why they'll make you worse

The various oral Diabetes medications described in Chapter Five are effective at lowering blood sugar and therefore reducing the risk of diabetic complications. Unfortunately many type 2 diabetics would not need these medications if they followed an appropriate eating plan, had a healthy lifestyle and took specific supplements to help control their blood sugar.

People in the early stages of Type 2 Diabetes are typically told to make changes to their diet and start exercising in order to get their blood sugar down. We say these people have "diet controlled" Diabetes, meaning they do not take any medication for the condition. Unfortunately in most cases these attempts are not successful and the majority of people eventually need to start taking tablets in order to control their blood sugar.

The standard recommendation for diabetics is to follow a low fat, high carbohydrate diet. Unfortunately this makes most diabetics worse. People with Diabetes become frustrated because they believe they are doing the right thing yet still can't get their blood sugar down and still can't lose weight! In this section we will explain why we disagree with many of the dietary recommendations given to diabetics.

The diet advice you've been given and why it's making you worse

You should base your diet on carbohydrate rich foods

Diabetics are told to eat carbohydrate rich foods at every meal and snack; these include food like bread, pasta, rice, breakfast cereals and starchy vegetables such as potatoes and sweet potatoes.

Why it will make you worse

This recommendation is based on the belief that a low fat, high carbohydrate diet is the best way to lose weight. You are told that carbohydrates are good for you because they are very low in fat and contain no cholesterol, therefore they won't promote weight gain or the development of heart disease.

Carbohydrates are all digested into sugar; all of them eventually end up as glucose in your bloodstream. The rise in blood sugar they cause promotes the release of insulin. As you know, most type 2 diabetics are insulin resistant, meaning they already have too much insulin in their body which isn't working properly anymore. Increasing their insulin level even further will worsen the Diabetes.

Insulin promotes your body to store fat, inhibits your body from burning fat, encourages your liver to manufacture more cholesterol and trigylcerides, and makes you hungry; all working together to make the Diabetes worse. High insulin levels also promote the development of fatty liver disease. Eating more carbohydrate rich foods raises your blood sugar level which increases your need for Diabetes medication – either oral tablets or insulin. Increasing your dose of medication is usually a sign that a disease is getting worse. Base your diet on carbohydrate rich foods and your Diabetes will get worse.

Please note that it is possible to follow a high carbohydrate, low fat diet and achieve an improvement in Type 2 Diabetes *if* that diet causes you to lose weight and keep it off! The problem is most diabetics are not able to stick to such a diet because it makes them hungry and gives them cravings for sugary or high carbohydrate foods.

You must lose weight

Diabetics are always being told how important it is they lose weight and this is very true. Having extra fat around your abdomen promotes insulin resistance and results in poor blood sugar control. The problem is it is virtually impossible for most diabetics to lose a significant amount of weight while following a high carbohydrate diet. This is because they are already insulin resistant and carbohydrates promote more weight gain, as described in the previous point.

It is OK to eat small amounts of sugar

Diabetics are commonly told that small amounts of table sugar are okay to include in their diet.

Why it will make you worse

If you are already eating carbohydrate at each meal like you are told to do and your blood sugar is higher than 99mg/dL (5.5 mmol/L) fasting - you don't need more sugar, it will only make your Diabetes worse. **If you want to reverse Type 2 Diabetes you must reduce the carbohydrate content of your diet.**

You should base your diet on low GI foods

This is correct, but what you aren't told is that vegetables, salads, fish, chicken, meat, eggs and most dairy products are some of the lowest GI foods. Meat, fish, chicken and eggs have such a low GI that it's zero! Salad vegetables have a much lower GI than sweet potato and rye bread. The GI only measures how fast a food raises your blood glucose. If you want to lower your blood sugar and reverse Type 2 Diabetes you must reduce the total carbohydrate content of your diet. Some processed foods promoted as having a low GI are actually high in added sugar; read food labels carefully.

You shouldn't eat too much protein because it will damage your kidneys

Because diabetics are prone to developing kidney disease, they are told to keep their intake of protein low because it may "over work" their kidneys.

Why this is untrue

We are not advocating diabetics eat loads of protein, just protein at each meal because it keeps your blood sugar stable and keeps you feeling full and satisfied. Healthy people who eat lots of protein don't get kidney disease; the main cause of kidney disease in diabetics is high blood sugar and high blood pressure. If you already have kidney damage you may need to follow a low protein diet, but protein won't damage your kidneys if they are currently healthy.

You should avoid fat and severely restrict eggs and red meat in your diet

Diabetics are consistently told to restrict their intake of all fat and cholesterol containing foods.

Why this is unnecessary

Diabetics are told to avoid these foods because of the mistaken belief they cause weight gain, clogged arteries and cardiovascular disease. You will gain weight a lot faster by eating bread, pasta, rice and potatoes than eating eggs and red meat. Eating foods that contain cholesterol has a negligible effect on your blood cholesterol level. The majority of the cholesterol in your body was made by your liver. The best way to bring your cholesterol down is to improve your liver health and reduce your blood insulin level, which will reduce the amount of cholesterol your liver manufactures.

Please avoid eating low fat foods. Compare a low fat food with its regular counterpart in a supermarket; nine times out of ten the low fat food will be higher in carbohydrate and/or sugar.

There is no cure for Type 2 Diabetes

If you follow an appropriate low carbohydrate eating plan, exercise and have a healthy lifestyle you have an excellent chance of getting your blood sugar down into the normal range; therefore would no longer be considered a diabetic. Type 2 Diabetes can be reversed and managed if you consistently follow a healthy diet and lifestyle.

8. Reversing Type 2 Diabetes through lifestyle changes

Following a healthy low carbohydrate diet is essential for diabetics, but so too is a healthy lifestyle. It is often unhealthy lifestyle habits that lead to poor food choices and promote Diabetes or worsen the disease when it is already present. This chapter will focus on exercise, stress and sleep as ways of maintaining healthy blood glucose levels, keeping your weight down and avoiding the long term complications of Diabetes.

The importance of exercise

Being overweight is the biggest risk factor for developing Type 2 Diabetes and weight loss is an excellent way to improve insulin sensitivity. Regular exercise is an effective way to keep your weight down and prevent developing Diabetes in the first place, but it is also essential in order to reverse Type 2 Diabetes because it can lower blood sugar.

Exercise helps diabetics in several important ways:

• Exercise lowers the rise in blood sugar that occurs after a meal. This is when blood sugar gets highest and causes most damage to your body. Therefore exercise reduces your risk of diabetic complications.

• Exercise lowers HbA1c.

• Exercise lowers blood pressure.

• It increases your body's sensitivity to insulin, thereby helping to prevent or reverse insulin resistance.

• Exercise lowers triglycerides and LDL "bad" cholesterol and raises HDL "good" cholesterol. In this way exercise helps to prevent heart disease.

• It increases energy levels and motivation to follow a healthy diet.

• It improves circulation and boosts your immune system's ability to fight infections.

- Exercise helps to prevent depression and it has a calming effect.

- Regular exercise promotes sound sleep.

What happens while you exercise?

When you exercise, your muscles require energy in the form of glucose. Some glucose is stored in your muscles and it will be used up. If you continue to exercise, your muscles will require more glucose; this is supplied by the glucose stored in your liver and also fat deposits, which are converted into glucose and burnt off. In this way exercise lowers your blood sugar level. Diabetics should not perform very intense exercise if they are not fit because this can actually raise their blood sugar. Intense exercise is a stress on your body and it stimulates the release of stress hormones such as adrenalin, which have a blood sugar elevating effect.

The best types of exercise for diabetics

Ideally you should exercise every day for 20 to 40 minutes. If you can't fit it in every day then aim for five days a week. The two main types of exercise are aerobic exercise and strength training. Aerobic exercise is something that makes you huff and puff, raises your heart rate and makes you break into a sweat. Examples of aerobic exercise are walking, jogging, cycling, swimming, dancing, tennis and other fast paced sports. This type of exercise is excellent for weight loss and improving the health of your heart. This type of exercise is more likely to cause Hypoglycemia (low blood sugar) in a diabetic than strength training.

Strength training is exercise that involves the use of weights that act as resistance, or your own body weight can act as resistance. This type of exercise is usually carried out at a gym, or can be done with equipment in your home. Hand weights are easily purchased from sports shops and department stores, or you could use canned food tins or other heavy objects in your home. Exercises that use your own body weight as resistance include push ups, triceps dips, squats and lunges. To increase the workload when you get stronger you can hold on to heavy objects while you do squats and lunges.

Strength training is excellent at improving your muscle cells' sensitivity to insulin, thereby helping insulin levels and blood sugar levels to come down. A US study recruited 22 overweight teenage boys; half of the group performed weight lifting workouts twice a week for 16 weeks and the other half did no exercise. After the 16 weeks the boys who exercised experienced gains in upper body and lower body strength. These boys experienced an improvement in insulin sensitivity of 45 percent! Interestingly, the boys who did no exercise experienced a fall in insulin sensitivity of one percent! This just shows that if you do no exercise, you will continue to become more insulin resistant and your blood sugar level will gradually rise.

Important points to remember

To help keep your blood sugar stable and reduce the risk of Hypoglycemia, make sure you test your blood sugar regularly so that you are aware what effect exercise has on you. It is also useful to be consistent with your meals, snacks, medication and exercise routine and do these things at the same time each day.

Sleep

A lack of quality sleep places you at increased risk of several health problems. If you are a diabetic it will make weight loss and blood sugar control much harder. Regularly not getting enough sleep makes your body less sensitive to insulin, therefore places you at increased risk of weight gain, high blood pressure and Syndrome X. Regularly getting 6.5 or less hours of sleep per night triggers a hormonal imbalance in your body that affects your appetite and behavior.

If you are tired through lack of sleep, you will experience more hunger; you are likely to crave unhealthy foods and you are less likely to exercise. People who don't get enough sleep have lower blood levels of the hormone leptin. Leptin is secreted by fat cells and acts to suppress appetite and lets the brain know that the body is well nourished and has enough fat stores. Sleep deprivation also raises blood levels of grehlin; a hormone released by the stomach that increases hunger. Therefore the more sleep deprived you are, the hungrier you will be.

This pattern is especially prevalent in children and young adults; the effect tends to drop off as we get older. If you are tired and hungry you are far less likely to make healthy food choices. Whatever is fastest and easiest is the most tempting option. Preparing healthy food from scratch seems far too hard and laborious. You are especially likely to crave sugary or salty snacks that are easy to eat and require no preparation. Eating sugar will give your blood sugar level a spike, providing a temporary boost in energy, but this is very short lived. You are also not likely to be motivated to exercise if you're feeling tired and drowsy.

Unfortunately, many of the harmful effects of sleep deprivation also affect people who work during the night and sleep during the day. If you do not sleep in complete darkness the pineal gland in your brain will not be able to produce sufficient quantities of the hormone melatonin, which is responsible for ensuring a deep sleep. Ideally you would get seven to nine hours of good sleep each night. If that's not happening at the moment, or you are a restless sleeper who wakes frequently, here are some tips for getting a better night's sleep:

Tips for better quality sleep

• If you suffer with insomnia find out the reason for it. Sometimes the reason is obvious, such as grief, financial problems and relationship difficulties, but other times the reason is not apparent. The book *Tired of Not Sleeping* explains 68 possible causes of insomnia and offers solutions for them.

• Try to get to bed roughly the same time each night and avoid staying up too late. Organise your time well so that you are not struggling to get things done late at night. The hours of sleep before 12am are said to be most therapeutic for the body.

• Perform a relaxing activity before bed such as reading a book, having a bath or having sex. Avoid mentally stimulating activities like using the internet, watching dramatic television shows or playing computer games.

• Avoid eating too late in the evening. It is especially important to avoid high carbohydrate foods, as they can cause an unstable blood sugar level at night, promoting a restless sleep. Eating oily or spicy food can promote heartburn, which obviously inhibits good sleep.

• Magnesium is often called "the great relaxer" because of the calming effect it has on the nervous system and muscles. Take a dose of magnesium with lunch and another one with dinner to improve the quality of your sleep.

• Sometimes depression can be responsible for insomnia or poor quality of sleep. If this is the case for you make sure you get 30 minutes of exercise most days of the week and try to go outside and get some sunlight several times a week. Fish oil is a great source of omega 3 fats, which have been proven to fight depression. St. John's Wort is an effective herb for depression but it cannot be taken by people on certain medications. St. John's Wort works best when combined with minerals and B vitamins. Depression is covered in more detail later on in this chapter.

Try to sleep in complete darkness and do not turn the light on if you get up to use the bathroom. Exposure to light during the night will disrupt production of melatonin by your pineal gland. See the book *Tired of Not Sleeping* for more information about overcoming insomnia.

Stress management

Stress has many harmful effects on your health. It increases your chances of developing Type 2 Diabetes and will make the disease worse if you already have it. Studies have shown that intense stress in middle age, such as death of a loved one or financial crisis significantly increases the risk of Diabetes even if a person has no family history of the disease. Ongoing work related stress also increases the risk of Diabetes.

Diabetics who experience chronic or intense stress find it much harder to keep their blood sugar down. The hormones adrenalin and cortisol that your body produces when stressed have a blood sugar elevating effect. Stress often causes people to eat poorly, skip meals and it can even make you forget to take your medication. Feeling overwhelmed and out of control can make healthy food preparation seem impossible.

You can't eliminate all stress from your life, and you wouldn't want to because it is a driving force that motivates us to get things done.

To reduce the stress in your life you need to either change the circumstances you are in or change your view of them. Here are some tips on keeping your stress levels down:

• **Take time out to relax:** It is vitally important to spend some quiet time devoted to a relaxing activity you enjoy. This may be something like listening to your favorite music, reading a good novel, meditation, yoga or deep breathing exercises.

• **Be kind to yourself:** Listen to the way you speak to yourself in your head. Do you treat yourself like a dear friend or an enemy? Sometimes we expect too much of ourselves and try to live up to perfect standards. It is okay to let go of too high standards.

• **Exercise:** Treat exercise as time out for yourself when you can take a break from your everyday hassles. Exercise causes your brain to release endorphins that have a calming and mood elevating effect.

• **Talk to someone:** Don't keep your problems and fears bottled up inside. Having a confidante that listens to your concerns can help to lessen any problem. Alternatively, you could speak to a counsellor or psychologist.

• **Accept what you have no control over:** Realize that there are some circumstances that you really have no control over and it is a waste of energy even trying. Remember too that you cannot control other people, only yourself.

Coping with depression

Depression is thought to be twice as common in diabetics as the general population. Being depressed can greatly hinder your ability to stick with a healthy eating plan, cope with dietary restrictions and it lowers your motivation to take care of yourself. People with depression develop more diabetic complications.

How do you know if you are depressed?

The symptoms of depression can creep on slowly, so that you are not aware you are affected. The most common symptoms of depression include the following:

- Sadness

- Anxiety

- Irritability

- Insomnia – inability to fall asleep or waking frequently or waking early

- Feelings of guilt and inadequacy

- Inability to concentrate

- Loss of interest in activities usually enjoyed

- Withdrawal from social activities

- Change in appetite – either loss of appetite or wanting to eat all the time

- Fatigue including physical and mental sluggishness

- Thoughts of death or suicide

There is no laboratory test to diagnose depression; it is diagnosed on the basis of symptoms.

Treatment of depression

The treatment of depression ideally includes both physical and emotional support. The following factors are all helpful in overcoming depression:

• **Make sure your diet is as healthy as possible.** Sugar and high carbohydrate foods can cause mood swings, anxiety and depression. If you follow our eating plan in Chapter Eleven you can reverse your Diabetes and improve your mood.

• **Include plenty of omega 3 fats in your diet.** A great deal of research has shown that omega 3 fats help to prevent and treat mild to moderate depression. The best source of these fats is seafood, especially sardines, mackerel, pilchards, wild salmon and anchovies. Omega 3 fats are found in smaller quantities in flaxseeds and walnuts. If you have depression you should take a fish oil supplement to increase your body's level of omega 3 fats faster.

• **Go outside and get some sunshine several times a week.** When sunshine hits our skin the cholesterol in our skin is converted into vitamin D. This vitamin has known mood elevating effects.

• **Do aerobic exercise for at least 30 minutes** a minimum of three times a week. Exercise that raises your heart rate and makes you sweat is an essential part of the treatment of depression.

• **Speaking to a counsellor, psychologist or psychotherapist** is an effective way of getting to the bottom of why you are depressed and modifying your thinking.

• **Magnesium and the herb St. John's Wort** (Hypericum) are very helpful in the treatment of depression. Magnesium helps to physically relax your body and helps you to cope with stress. It can help to relieve muscle tension and promotes a better night's sleep. St. John's Wort has been clinically proven to help with mild to moderate depression. This herb cannot be taken with prescription antidepressant medication and it interacts with many other prescription drugs. Please consult your health care practitioner if you wish to take it.

• **In some cases a prescription antidepressant medication is required.** There are several options and your doctor can help you find one that effectively treats your depression and has minimal side effects. The book Tired of not Sleeping contains more information about the use of antidepressant medication.

9. Reversing Type 2 Diabetes through nutritional and herbal medicine

Having a healthy diet and lifestyle are the most important factors in preventing or reversing Type 2 Diabetes. However there are a number of herbs, vitamins and minerals that have been shown to help diabetics. Studies have found they can help to control blood sugar levels and improve insulin sensitivity, as well as help prevent the complications of Diabetes. In addition, people who are deficient in certain nutrients are at much greater risk of developing Type 2 Diabetes in the first place.

Research conducted in the United States found that diabetics who take nutritional supplements (roughly 34 percent of diabetics) are more likely to report that they are in good to excellent health. Diabetics who don't take nutritional supplements typically rate their health as fair or poor. If you combine a healthy diet and lifestyle with the right supplements, you have the best chance of reversing Type 2 Diabetes.

Helpful Supplements for Diabetics

• Gymnema Sylvestre

According to several human clinical trials the action of the herb Gymnema Sylvestre can be beneficial in those with elevated blood glucose levels. High blood levels of glucose (hyperglycemia), high cholesterol and excessive glycosylation of proteins, appear to be corrected by Gymnema Sylvestre. It is postulated that the beneficial action of this herb works by regenerating damaged beta cells in the pancreas. The beta cells produce insulin and are often damaged in diabetics. Gymnema also reduces cravings for sugar and refined carbohydrates.

Clinical trials of Gymnema Sylvestre used an equivalent of 400mg daily of the whole herb from a 5:1 extract of Gymnema Sylvestre.[27]

• Bitter Melon

The herb Bitter Melon is also known as Momordica Charantia, or bitter gourd. The fruit of this plant is a popular food in India. Clinical trials and laboratory experiments using an extract of the dried fruit or ground seeds of Bitter Melon, revealed its ability to lower blood glucose levels. These studies found that Bitter Melon is an effective hypoglycemic agent that reduces excessive blood glucose levels in Type 2 Diabetics. The recommended daily dosage of Bitter Melon is an equivalent of 5 grams of the fruit powder using an 8:1 standardized extract.[27A]

• Chromium picolinate

Chromium is required for the healthy function of the insulin receptors, which are situated on the surface of the cells. This is very important for those with insulin resistance where the receptors malfunction, and become resistant to the action of insulin. In other words chromium helps the cells to communicate better with the insulin hormone, thereby facilitating the transfer of glucose from the blood stream into the cell. Deficiency of chromium is common in those who have consumed a diet high in refined carbohydrates. It is difficult to get all the chromium you need from your diet, as the richest sources are Brewer's yeast and liver.

Chromium is a vital component of Glucose Tolerance Factor (GTF) which improves insulin function. Those who are deficient in chromium have difficulty in regulating blood glucose levels.

Chromium picolinate has been shown to reduce insulin resistance, lower blood glucose levels by 18%, and glycosylated hemoglobin (HgbA1c) by 10%.[27B]

Chromium picolinate is a bioactive source of this essential mineral. The efficiency of chromium absorption is very low, but the picolinic acid in the Chromium Picolinate form is a mineral transporter, which transports chromium into the muscle. Chromium picolinate is an excellent supplement for sports people and diabetics.

Results from a study in Beijing by Anderson et al., indicate that chromium may be efficacious in treating Type 2 Diabetes. The metabolic effects of chromium picolinate in this large study were comparable to oral hypoglycemic agents or insulin.

• Lipoic Acid

Lipoic acid is a natural substance, which has been demonstrated to be effective in improving glucose utilization and reducing the glycosylation of proteins. Improving the utilization of glucose will contribute a great deal towards preventing the complications of diabetes such as hypertension, kidney failure, heart disease, cataracts, macular degeneration and severe nerve damage.

Lipoic acid has repeatedly been shown to counteract insulin resistance in muscle tissue, and this is the major mechanism whereby it effectively lowers blood glucose levels. The potent antioxidant action of lipoic acid may be very useful in slowing the development of diabetic cataracts and neuropathy. Doses of lipoic acid range from 100 to 600mg daily.[28]

• Carnitine fumarate

Carnitine is a natural substance made in the body from the amino acids lysine and methionine. Carnitine is involved in fat mobilization, and when it is deficient, overweight persons often find it very difficult to get into the fat burning area of metabolism. In other words, they have difficulty beginning the breakdown of body fat, which is called the stage of lipolysis and ketosis. Carnitine can be described as the "shovel" that puts the fuel into the energy factories (mitochondria) inside the cells to be converted to energy.[29] The richest dietary sources of carnitine are red meats (lamb and beef).

• Selenium and other minerals

Selenium should be supplemented in diabetics, because of its potent antioxidant and protective effects.[30]

Magnesium, manganese and zinc are involved in multiple enzyme systems within the energy producing mitochondria. A diet high in carbohydrates, especially of the refined types, may cause depletion of trace minerals such as manganese, selenium and zinc, which will slow down metabolism.

Magnesium has been shown to reduce insulin resistance and if you are diabetic, I highly recommend that you take supplemental magnesium. Taking 400mg of supplemental magnesium each day has been shown to improve blood sugar control.[32]

Magnesium is essential for other reasons; it helps to reduce high blood pressure and cardiovascular disease. Diabetics lose greater amounts of magnesium in their urine than healthy people, therefore a supplement is strongly recommended to prevent a deficiency.

Mineral deficiencies are common in diabetics and will worsen glucose intolerance.[31]

The nutrients discussed above are helpful for -

- Insulin resistance
- Unstable blood glucose levels including high blood glucose levels (hyperglycemia) and low blood glucose levels (hypoglycemia)
- Cravings for sugar and high GI carbohydrates
- Weight excess in those with impaired glucose tolerance

Suitable doses are shown below -

- Gymnema Sylvestre (5:1 standardized extract) 27.0mg equiv. to 133.3mg
- Bitter melon (8:1 standardized extract) 208.3mg equiv. to 1666.7mg
- Chromium picolinate 134mcg
- Lipoic acid 70mg
- Carnitine fumarate 150mg
- Selenomethionine 8.6mcg
- Magnesium aspartate 16.7mg
- Manganese chelate 3.3mg
- Zinc chelate 1.33mg
- Vitamin E 20i.u.

All these supplements may be taken individually or combined together in Glicemic Balance capsules.

Take two to four capsules of **Glicemic Balance** daily.

These supplements will not interact adversely with insulin or oral hypoglycemic drugs. However you should be guided by your own doctor. If you need more information on supplements or diet, phone 623 334 3232 in the USA or 02 4655 8855 in Australia.

Precautions while using natural supplements

Insulin dependent diabetics must not stop their insulin medication Diabetics on oral hypoglycemic drugs can only stop their medication with their own doctor's approval. Those taking the above supplements for the first time may notice that their blood glucose levels drop excessively, and this can be avoided by eating at least three regular meals daily, with every meal containing first class protein. Healthy in between meal snacks may also be required, consisting of nuts, seeds, sardines, tuna, crabmeat, salads or protein powder.

• Cinnamon

Cinnamon is one of the oldest used remedies in Chinese medicine. It has numerous benefits, including blood thinning, antimicrobial actions and blood sugar control. Research has shown that cinnamon can lower fasting glucose levels. A therapeutic dose of cinnamon is between 1 and 6 grams a day; doses in this range can reduce fasting glucose by 18-29 percent, if taken for 40 days. You can include cinnamon in your diet or take it in supplement form. Cinnamon can be used in smoothies or stewed fruit.

• Fenugreek

Fenugreek seeds are commonly used as a spice in Indian and Thai cooking. They have the ability to lower blood glucose levels in Type 2 Diabetics. Taking 15 grams per day of ground fenugreek can reduce blood glucose levels after a meal.[28] Fenugreek has a very strong odor but you can obtain odor free concentrated extracts in supplement form and a dose as low as one gram per day can improve blood sugar control and Syndrome X.[32] Fenugreek tea is available from health food stores, but please be aware that your body may emit an odor the day after drinking it!

Watch your iron level

It is well known that iron deficiency causes anemia, but too much iron can cause even more problems. Research published in the journal Diabetes Care has found that diabetic women with the highest blood iron levels have a 50 percent higher risk of heart disease than women with the lowest iron levels, especially if they are postmenopausal. Researchers followed 6,161 type 2 diabetic women from the Nurses' Health Study for 20 years to arrive at this conclusion.[33] Previous research has shown that men with high iron levels are more prone to heart disease too. If you are a diabetic it is advisable to have your iron level checked with a blood test regularly. If it is high, blood donations are an effective way to reduce iron.

Antioxidants

A high intake of antioxidants in your diet can help to protect you from developing Type 2 Diabetes and will improve your outcome if you already have the disease. Antioxidants are substances that scavenge free radicals; these are damaging compounds found in the body that can damage your cell membranes, DNA (genetic material) and even cause cell death. Free radicals are generated in many ways; they come from environmental pollution and cigarette smoke, from your diet if you eat fats that have been damaged by frying, or nitrates in preserved meat like bacon, ham and small goods. However, a large number of free radicals are generated within your own body as a result of normal metabolic processes such as digestion, energy production, detoxification and immune system reactions.

Diabetics are known to have a great deal of inflammation constantly occurring in their body. This is primarily a result of having a high blood sugar level and excess fat on their body. Fat cells (adipocytes) produce a whole range of chemicals that create inflammation and free radical damage in your body; these same chemicals are made by your immune system. If you have a lot of extra fat on your body, your fat cells will be pumping out great quantities of chemicals that cause tissue damage and inflammation. The sticky nature of sugar causes it to create a lot of tissue damage also, which your body constantly tries to repair. Free radical damage in a diabetic's body is a leading cause of complications of the disease and it speeds up the rate of aging.

Diabetics use up antioxidants at a much faster rate trying to repair this damage. If you are a diabetic you have a much greater requirement for antioxidants and it is essential you get enough in your diet. This is an important way to avoid or delay the development of diabetic complications, such as neuropathy, blood vessel disease and retinopathy. Antioxidants will also boost your immune system and reduce your risk of infections.

The best source of antioxidants

Antioxidants are usually the substances that give food its color; such as in fruit and vegetables and red wine. That's why it is important to eat a wide variety of fresh produce, so that you will obtain as many antioxidants as possible. Many people stick to the same fruit and vegetables each day. There are probably vegetables in your local grocery store you have never tasted and don't know how to prepare. Experiment with as many fresh foods as possible to keep your diet varied and nutrient filled.

An interesting study was published in the *American Journal of Clinical Nutrition*. Researchers ana lysed 1113 commonly eaten foods in the USA with the aim of ranking them in a table of highest antioxidant content to lowest.[34] They found that the food groups with greatest antioxidant content are spices and herbs, nuts and seeds, berries and fruit and vegetables. From the 50 foods that ranked highest in antioxidants, 13 were spices, 8 were fruits or vegetables, 5 were berries, 5 were breakfast cereals, 5 were chocolate based, and 4 were nuts and seeds. When you take typical serving sizes into account, the foods that ranked highest are: blackberries, walnuts, strawberries, artichokes, cranberries, brewed coffee, raspberries, pecans, blueberries, ground cloves, grape juice and unsweetened baking chocolate. Previous studies have found that blueberries actually come out on top; so it is probably best to assume that all berries are some of the highest antioxidant containing foods.

Glicemic Balance capsules contain an effective dose of the herbs

Gymnema Sylvestre and Bitter Melon combined with chromium picolinate, selenium, magnesium, zinc, manganese, lipoic acid and carnitine. It is recommended to take one or two capsules, three times daily with meals.

Table of antioxidant content of some of the top foods

FOOD	ANTIOXIDANT CONTENT in mmol/100g
Blackberries	5.75
Walnuts	3.72
Strawberries	3.58
Artichokes, cooked	3.56
Cranberries	3.13
Raspberries	2.87
Blueberries	2.68
Cloves, ground	2.64
Prunes	1.72
Cabbage, red, cooked	1.61
Pineapple	1.28
Oranges	1.26
Plums, black	1.21
Pinto beans	1.14
Spinach	1.05
Kiwi fruit	0.99
Tea, brewed	0.88
Red bell pepper	0.82

Dark chocolate is an excellent source of antioxidants if it contains at least 70 percent cocoa solids. The only problem with chocolate is its sugar content, which should be avoided if you have high blood sugar. Sugar free chocolate is now available in health food stores and supermarkets. Alternatively, you can make a hot chocolate drink by combining unsweetened baking cocoa, stevia and hot water.

Red wine contains powerful antioxidants too, but it is best avoided if you are trying to reduce your blood sugar level.

10. Specific recommendations for avoiding diabetic complications

The main way to avoid developing the complications or consequences of Diabetes is to keep your blood sugar level as close to normal as possible and keep your weight in the healthy range. However, there are specific nutrients that are effective at preventing or minimizing the impact of diabetic complications. This section will give you a summary of recommendations for each condition.

Cardiovascular disease:

• Avoid sugar and follow an eating plan that is lower in carbohydrate and higher in protein. Eat more fiber from foods such as vegetables, nuts, seeds, legumes and fruit. This will help to keep your weight in a healthy range and will keep your blood fats (cholesterol, triglycerides) in the normal range.

• Exercise regularly, including a mix of aerobic and strength training exercise.

• Take an omega 3 fish oil supplement at a dose of 3 to 6 capsules per day.

• Take the antioxidant nutrients selenium, vitamin E and vitamin C, which help to protect the cholesterol in your body from becoming oxidized and causing damage to your arteries. You can find these nutrients combined in tablet form.

• Regularly consume garlic, onion, ginger and turmeric, as they have blood thinning and antioxidant properties.

• See our book Cholesterol the Real Truth for in-depth information on how to reduce your risk of heart attacks and strokes. The recommendations in this book will also help if you have high blood pressure.

Diabetic eye disease:

Losing your sight is a devastating effect of Diabetes. Along with our diet recommendations in Chapter Eleven, please ensure you do the following:

• Take a supplement containing bilberry extract at a dose of 160 to 320 mg per day. Bilberry is extremely high in antioxidants that have a special affinity for the eyes and can protect them from free radical damage.

• The carotenoid antioxidants lutein, lycopene and zeaxanthin all help to protect your eyes from diseases including cataracts, glaucoma, retinopathy and age related macula degeneration. They are found in dark green leafy vegetables such as spinach and Asian leafy greens, as well as brightly colored orange and red fruits and vegetables such as tomatoes, sweet potatoes, carrots, pumpkin, bell pepper and mangoes. You absorb carotenoids from foods much better if you eat some fat at the same meal, for example olive oil or avocado. Egg yolks are an excellent source of the antioxidant zeaxanthin, so please eat more of them.

• Raw vegetable juices are an excellent source of antioxidants; however they can be high in sugar, depending on which vegetables are used. A beneficial juice for eye disease contains ¼ of a beet, 1 small carrot, 20 green beans and 1 bell pepper. **All diabetics must avoid fruit juice.**

• Omega 3 fats are anti inflammatory and can help to protect your vision. Taking a fish oil supplement is recommended.

Diabetic kidney disease (nephropathy):

To protect your kidneys it is vital to keep your blood sugar level as close to normal as possible and to avoid high blood pressure. You should be able to achieve these goals by following our diet recommendations in Chapter Eleven. If you already have nephropathy and your kidney function is below 40 percent of normal, do not take any nutritional supplements unless you consult your doctor first.

Diabetic nerve disease (neuropathy):

• Lipoic acid at a dose of 600 to 1800mg daily should give symptom relief if taken for several months.

• The cholesterol lowering drugs called statins can cause neuropathy, along with a host of other side effects. Examples of statins are Lipitor, Pravachol, Zocor and Lipex. Speak to your doctor about coming off these drugs if you take them and have neuropathy. Our book Cholesterol the Real Truth gives you a treatment plan to lower your cholesterol.

• Ensure you have plenty of beneficial fats in your diet, as fat provides a protective coating around your nerves and facilitates their function. You can find beneficial fatty acids in fish, olive oil, avocados, raw nuts and seeds, whole eggs, ground flaxseeds and virgin organic coconut oil.

Infections:

Sugar suppresses your immune system and encourages the growth of bacteria and fungi; so the ultimate way to reduce your risk of infections is to keep your blood sugar within normal limits and avoid sugar in your diet.

• Include plenty of antioxidants in your diet, as they act to boost your immune system. See Chapter Nine for information about antioxidants.

• Try to control your stress level, as stress is enormously draining on your immune system.

• Avoid all dairy products if you have a respiratory infection such as bronchitis, sinusitis or an ear infection. Dairy products increase congestion and mucus production.

• Many herbs, spices and foods have anti viral properties. Include as many of these as possible in your diet. Some of these include garlic, onion, mushrooms, cabbage, fresh coconut, thyme, radish, ginger root, lemon, oregano, chili, grapefruit and walnuts.

• Skin infections are very common in diabetics especially with the gram positive bacteria staphylococcus and streptococcus. This can range from small red pimples to blisters, deep abscesses and cellulitis. To prevent these potentially serious problems I highly reccommend that you use tea tree oil soap and/or tea tree body wash every day all over your body.

• Olive leaf has antiviral and anti microbial properties and helps your body to fight infections.

• Selenium can inhibit the replication of viruses in your body; it is often known as the "viral birth control pill". Selenium can strengthen the immune system against most kinds of infections and supports healing of injured tissues. Selenium works best when combined with vitamin E, zinc and vitamin C.

Please phone our Health Advisory Service in Australia on 02 4655 8855 or 623 334 3232 in the USA and speak to a naturopath if you need more information.

Erectile dysfunction:

Men who are slim and fit are much less likely to develop this condition. The health of the arteries in your penis is an indicator of the health of the arteries in your heart. Erectile dysfunction is often an early warning sign of cardiovascular disease. If you have started to experience erectile problems it is essential to improve your diet and lifestyle now, before damage to the nerves and blood vessels in your penis is irreversible. Diabetes and obesity cause a decline in your testosterone level, which will improve when you reverse these conditions. To overcome erectile dysfunction, please follow our eating plan in Chapter Eleven and the suggestions for cardiovascular disease and neuropathy in this chapter.

11. Eating plan to reverse type 2 Diabetes

Guidelines for the Eating Plan

Below you will find lists of foods that are allowed, and which foods you must avoid. These are the basic rules of the eating plan. The best choices are the foods that are lowest in carbohydrate, and the rest are higher in carbohydrate but still acceptable. You are free to make up your own meals out of the foods listed here, or if you like you can follow the recipes that we have provided. If cooking is a chore for you and you don't mind eating simple food, then just eat according to the lists below. However, if you get bored easily, or want new ideas for low carbohydrate meals, you will find our recipes interesting and tasty.

Foods you can eat

Protein

Meat	Seafood	Poultry	Eggs
Beef	Fresh/Tinned Fish	Chicken (no stuffing)	Boiled
Veal	Prawns	Duck	Poached
Lamb	Lobster	Quail	Omelet
Pork	Crab	Turkey	Scrambled
Game meat	Oysters and Mussels	Goose	
Venison			

Meat should be purchased fresh. Avoid or minimize smoked meat, bacon, ham, sausages, hot dogs and other small goods because of the preservatives found in them which are carcinogenic.

Remember that offal, (kidney and liver etc.) oysters and muscles are higher in carbohydrate than other meat and seafood; they can be consumed but in smaller quantities.

Dairy products such as cheese and yogurt contain protein and you can eat them, but they should <u>not</u> be consumed in the same quantity as the other sources of protein listed because they are often high in carbohydrate and/or fat.

Vegetables

These vegetables are lowest in carbohydrate and are the ones you should eat most of. Please eat at least two cups of these vegetables daily.

Best Choice

- Radishes

- Celery

- Mushrooms

- Broccoli

- Kale

- Collards

- Cauliflower

- Fresh herbs – parsley, basil, cilantro, dill, watercress, rocket (arugula)

- Lettuce

- Cabbage

- Brussels sprouts

- Endive

- Chicory

- Green beans

- Bok choy and other leafy Asian vegetables

- Fennel

- Chilies
- Cucumber
- Asparagus
- Spinach
- Leek
- Ginger root and garlic

The Rest

These vegetables are allowed, but in smaller quantities because they are higher in carbohydrate.

- Zucchini
- Squash
- Turnip
- Bamboo shoots
- Kohl rabi
- Bell pepper
- Okra
- Aubergine
- Avocado
- Tomato
- Carrot
- Onion
- Pumpkin
- Beet

Vegetables to Avoid

Starchy vegetables must be avoided for now; these include potatoes, sweet potatoes, parsnip and Swedes. Remember that corn is a grain, and like all grains, it must be avoided.

Fruit

Fruit needs to be limited to not more than two servings per day. Fruit juices and dried fruit must be avoided.

Best Choices

These are the best fruits for diabetics because they contain specific fruit acids which help insulin to work in the body.

- Berries – strawberries, blueberries, raspberries, blackberries, mulberries, gooseberries

- Green apples

- Kiwi fruit

- Passionfruit

- Cherries

- Grapefruit, lemons and limes

- Tamarillos

All other fruits are allowed except for bananas and mangoes.

Nuts and Seeds

These are best eaten raw, not roasted. This is because the delicate essential fatty acids are easily damaged by roasting. Nuts and seeds are best eaten unsalted.

Best Choices

- Brazil nuts

- Sesame seeds

- Walnuts

- Almonds

- Pepitas (pumpkin seeds)

- Pecans

- Coconut

The Rest

- Macadamias
- Hazelnuts
- Sunflower seeds
- Cashews
- Pine nuts
- Peanuts
- Pistachios

Keep in mind that cashews are the nuts highest in carbohydrate, so keep your intake of these to a minimum. Peanuts are best avoided or minimized. You can have one heaped tablespoon of nut butter or nut paste per day. Make sure it contains no other ingredients except nuts.

Dairy Products

If you suffer with a condition such as eczema, hay fever, sinusitis, asthma, an auto immune condition or fluid retention, you are best avoiding dairy products. Goat, sheep and buffalo milk products are usually less allergenic and easier to digest than those made from cow's milk. Avoid drinking large quantities of milk, as the lactose in it makes it fairly high in carbohydrate.

Best Choices

- Plain full fat yogurt, quark or cottage cheese
- Feta cheese
- Parmesan cheese
- Pecorino cheese
- Romano cheese
- Ricotta

You can eat between 80 and 100 grams of cheese or yogurt per day.

Avoid fat reduced cheese. Skim milk is higher in carbohydrate than full fat milk, so if you use milk in tea or coffee you are better off using the full fat version.

Legumes

Small amounts of legumes are allowed because they offer many health benefits, but remember that they are all fairly high in carbohydrate. You need to limit your intake to not more than ½ cup of cooked legumes three times per week.

Best Choices

- Tofu
- Tempeh
- Green peas
- Soy beans

The Rest

- Chickpeas
- Kidney beans
- Lima beans
- Borlotti beans
- Adzuki beans
- Pinto beans
- Great Northern beans
- Navy beans
- Black beans
- Black-eyed beans
- Lentils
- Mung beans

- Baked beans need to be avoided because the sauce they are in usually contains sugar, which significantly raises their carbohydrate content.

Beverages

Best Choices

- Water; plain or with natural lemon or lime juice squeezed into it

- Soda water or mineral water

- Tea

- Coffee

- Herbal tea; as long as it is free of sugar and barley

Excessive caffeine can cause unstable blood sugar levels and promote insulin release; this can slow weight loss and stimulate cravings. Limit coffee to not more than 2 cups per day. If you drink decaffeinated coffee, make sure it is water decaffeinated. Herbal coffee substitutes that contain grains (e.g. Barley) must be avoided.

Alcohol

Most diabetics can drink small amounts of alcohol and still reverse their Diabetes. If you have a fatty liver or other liver disease it is best to avoid or minimize alcohol. If you are metabolically resistant (lose weight extremely slowly) it is also best to avoid alcohol. Diabetics should not drink alcohol on an empty stomach because it may lead to Hypoglycemia (low blood sugar). If you drink alcohol, do so with a meal.

If you are a man, do not have more than 2 standard drinks per day and have at least 3 alcohol free days per week. If you are a woman do not have more than 1 standard drink per day and have at least 3 alcohol free days per week.

Best Choices

- Spirits – vodka, gin, scotch, whisky

- Dry red wine

Spirits are best consumed either on the rocks, with water or soda water. Please avoid fruit juice, sugary drinks or diet soda as mixers.

Some people may get upset that alcohol is included, whilst others may breathe a sigh of relief. Indulge at your own risk if desired.

The most appropriate drinks are things like scotch and water with a splash of lemon or lime or vodka and soda water with some lemon or lime juice.

You can allow yourself a little cocktail night once a month. We have to learn to reward ourselves, I mean here you are, sticking to a new eating plan, doing everything in your power to heal yourself; you definitely need to reward your efforts. You can invite your friends over and just relax and unwind, the beneficial effects of which are highly under rated, yet truly recommended.

Freeing tension and stress, maybe having a couple of dances to your favorite tunes and investing in a night of laughs and fantasy; only you will truly be able to gauge the effects on your spirit. Please do not add into the equation a little hangover on the morning after; you are only allowed two cocktails, so sip slowly.

I am going to divulge a little cocktail recipe for you, but if you like this recipe you can keep your eyes out for our upcoming cocktail book called *Low Carb Cocktails to Lighten up Body, Mind and Spirit.*

Mixed Berry Delight

Ingredients

- 3 count pour of vodka (hold bottle upside down and count to 3)
- 4 fresh strawberries
- 6 fresh or frozen raspberries
- 2 fresh or frozen blackberries
- Pulp of 1 Passionfruit
- Juice of ½ a lime
- Juice of ¼ a lemon
- 8 drops liquid stevia
- 8 mint leaves
- ½ cup unsweetened berry juice

Method

- Put all ingredients into a blender with ice. Blend until smooth. Pour into a cocktail glass, garnish with a sprig of mint.

Herbs, Spices and Condiments

All herbs, spices and condiments are allowed as long as they do not contain sugar, or no more than 2 grams of carbohydrate per tablespoon. Fresh or dried herbs and spices are preferable to sauces, which are often high in sugar.

Best Choices

- Salt (sea salt or iodized sea salt is preferable)
- Pepper
- Cayenne
- Oregano
- Cilantro
- Garam masala
- Cumin
- Basil
- Thyme
- Cinnamon
- Chili
- Parsley
- Mint
- Sweet (Hungarian) paprika
- Curry powder
- Ginger root
- Garlic

- Olives
- Picked chilies
- Sun dried tomatoes
- Mustard
- Plain full fat yogurt
- Some mayonnaise – check the carbohydrate content
- Coconut milk

Fats and Oils

Best Choices

- Extra virgin olive oil
- Flaxseed (linseed) oil
- Macadamia oil
- Walnut oil
- Avocado oil
- Butter
- Ghee
- Organic virgin coconut oil. Avoid copha.

All oils must state they are cold pressed or extra virgin on the label. Olive oil, macadamia oil, butter, ghee and coconut oil can be used for cooking; the others can only be used cold over salads and vegetables.

Foods that must be avoided on the eating plan

All sugar, grains, cereals, starchy vegetables and high sugar fruits need to be avoided. All grains must be avoided, including wheat, rye, oats, barley, corn, rice, spelt, kamut, sorghum,amaranth, teff and quinoa. You must avoid all foods with flour in the ingredients list.

Foods to avoid include the following:

- Bread, including flat, unleavened bread
- Pasta
- Cereals
- Rice
- Noodles
- Pastry
- Cakes
- Cookies
- Crackers
- Corn
- Semolina
- Sago and tapioca
- Polenta
- Tortillas
- Potatoes
- Sweet potato
- Parsnips
- Swedes
- Bananas
- Mangoes
- Margarine
- Artificial sweeteners
- Sugar
- Honey
- Maple syrup
- Any food containing flour

Portion Sizes

It is far more relevant to focus on what you are eating rather than the quantity. You do not need to go hungry; it is possible to eat substantial, delicious, filling meals and still reduce your blood sugar and lose weight. You will find our diabetic eating plan easy to stick to because you should not be hungry. You will also find that your cravings will diminish.

At each meal, you must eat a serving of protein; that is lean meat, fish, chicken, whey protein powder or eggs. A serving is a palm and a half sized portion, or two eggs. You must have at least 2 cups of the "Best choice" vegetables from the list in this chapter and up to a cup daily of "The rest".

You are allowed up to two servings of fruit each day. For example, a serving may be one apple or four strawberries. Fresh fruit is preferable, but tinned fruit with no added sugar is acceptable. You can have up to a handful of raw nuts and seeds each day as snacks, or tossed into your salads. These need to be raw and not salted. You can include legumes in your diet up to three times a week; a serving is ½ cup of cooked legumes. It is important to include some good fats in your diet, as they will help to prevent you from feeling hungry, and reduce cravings. Good fats include a drizzle of olive or flaxseed oil on your salad or vegetables, ½ medium avocado daily, oily fish (such as salmon, trout, sardines, mackerel), raw nuts and seeds and coconut milk.

In the beginning avoiding sugar can be difficult, because of its addictive nature. Therefore, it is better to not worry about your portion sizes too much when starting out. Soon enough, as your insulin level falls, so too will your appetite and cravings.

You will have faster results in terms of weight loss if you drink approximately ten glasses of water each day. This can speed up your metabolic rate, flush toxins from your body, reduce appetite and help you to avoid constipation.

What about snacks?

Some diabetics need to have one or more snacks throughout the day to keep their blood sugar stable. That is fine as long as you choose a healthy snack from our list in the following section.

If you are not hungry between meals and your blood sugar level is stable, don't snack. Please use snacks only to satisfy hunger, not as a distraction from doing something unpleasant or as entertainment for your mouth! Try to keep busy, and fill your spare time with activities you enjoy. Please don't snack while performing other activities such as driving, ironing, watching television or using the computer. It is very easy to eat way more than you planned if your mind is occupied by something else. Whenever you eat, take the time to sit down, relax and really savor the taste of the food you are consuming. This way you will find it much more satisfying and be less likely to overeat.

Snack Ideas

You are most likely to succeed if you plan ahead of time. Prepare your snacks the night before and carry them with you the next day so that you are never in the situation that you're starving and there's nothing healthy to eat.

• A handful of nuts and/or seeds with a piece of fruit

• Hummus with vegetable sticks or tahini with vegetable sticks

• Plain yogurt with fresh berries, sweetened with stevia powder or liquid if desired

• Freshly cut apple segments spread with natural nut butter/paste

• A boiled egg with an apple

• Guacamole with vegetable sticks and nuts

• A piece of chicken, fish or meat with salad

• A whey protein powder smoothie

• A 1.5 inch slice of cheese with a piece of fruit

• Celery filled with Ricotta cheese or nut butter/paste

• Cottage cheese sprinkled with crushed walnuts

• Feta cheese sprinkled with dry roasted sesame seeds, served with cucumber and celery

Every snack must contain some protein; for example as found in nuts, seeds, legumes, whey protein powder, chicken, fish, eggs, dairy products or meat. Do not snack on fruit alone. Diabetics should not eat fruit on an empty stomach.

Avoiding Hypoglycemia (low blood sugar)

Hypoglycemia occurs when the blood sugar becomes too low; this is usually below 59 mg/dL (3.3 mmol/L). It is a very unpleasant experience but luckily there are ways you can avoid it.

Tips to prevent Hypoglycemia

- Eat regular meals. Don't go for long periods without eating.
- Avoid sudden changes in diet or exercise.
- Eat a snack before exercising.
- Always bring a suitable snack with you when travelling, such as some nuts and fruit.
- Always carry a small packet of jelly beans with you.

Symptoms of Hypoglycemia

- Hunger
- Weakness, shakiness or dizziness
- Headache
- Cold sweat and a clammy feeling
- Increased heart rate or pounding heart

Symptoms of more severe Hypoglycemia

- Confusion, irritability or nervousness
- Blurred vision or double vision
- Foggy brain
- Fainting spells
- Numbness or tingling in the fingers or lips

If not remedied, Hypoglycemia can get much worse and require urgent medical intervention.

Remedies to treat mild to moderate Hypoglycemia

- Have 6 jelly beans.

- If these are unavailable, you could have approximately 150mL (5 oz.) of fruit juice or soda pop.

Don't eat more than the suggested amount. Stop what you are doing and sit or lie down for ten to 15 minutes. If you don't feel better after that time have the same amount of food or drink again. After an episode of Hypoglycemia it is common to feel quite tired for several hours.

Eating out: your best options

Eating at restaurants is fairly easy because you can always order steak and salad, or chicken or fish and salad or cooked vegetables. Make sure you state that you do not want potatoes, as they usually come standard with restaurant meals.

Trying to find a healthy lunch in a shopping centre food court presents more of a challenge. Tuna salad or chicken salad is becoming more commonly available. If you really can't find anything to eat that doesn't involve bread or flour of some description, you can always go to a sandwich bar or delicatessen and request some salad and protein on a plate or in a box, as opposed to in a sandwich. So you would basically be eating the sandwich filling only.

Other ideas for meals when away from home are:

- Omelet

- Barbecued chicken with salad or vegetables

- Steak and salad

- Roast meat with salad or baked vegetables (other than potatoes)

- Grilled fish and salad

- Caesar salad (no croutons)

- Greek salad

- Seafood salad

- Poached eggs (no toast)

- Scrambled eggs (no toast)

- Frittata

- Shish kebab

Beware of sauces and dressings that may contain added sugar. Ask to have plain olive oil and vinegar as a salad dressing. Blue cheese or parmesan cheese can be sprinkled over steak as a dressing, as opposed to a sugar containing sauce or marinade.

Diabetic 2 week meal plan

This is a sample meal plan only to give you ideas. You can swap the meals around or modify the recipes, as long as you still follow the guidelines outlined in the beginning of this chapter.

Week 1

Monday

Breakfast:	Tomato frittata
Lunch:	Tuna salad with lime mayonnaise
Dinner:	Baked chicken breasts with lemon and feta, with a salad

Tuesday

Breakfast:	Strawberry delight smoothie
Lunch:	Chicken avocado salad
Dinner:	Middle Eastern fish

Wednesday

Breakfast:	Omelet with cheese, asparagus and mushrooms
Lunch:	Tasty lunchtime rissoles
Dinner:	Herb coated veal

Thursday

Breakfast:	Good morning squares
Lunch:	Warm bell pepper and zucchini with sardines
Dinner:	Chicken soup

Friday

Breakfast:	Peach and nut smoothie
Lunch:	Chicken and grapefruit salad
Dinner:	Salmon steaks with fennel

Saturday

Breakfast:	Mushroom frittata
Lunch:	Salmon and warm vegetable salad
Dinner:	Stir fried aubergine and tomatoes with lamb chops

Sunday

Breakfast:	Spinach omelet
Lunch:	Lemony chicken salad
Dinner:	Grilled salmon with avocado salsa

Week 2

Monday

Breakfast:	Quick and tasty egg breakfast
Lunch:	Chicken and blueberry salad
Dinner:	Veal cutlets

Tuesday

Breakfast:	Tropical smoothie
Lunch:	Sunflower salad with tuna
Dinner:	Chicken with olives

Wednesday

Breakfast:	Salmon omelet
Lunch:	Chicken and artichoke salad
Dinner:	Pork meatball soup

Thursday

Breakfast:	Low carb hash brown
Lunch:	Salmon salad
Dinner:	Gingery chicken

Friday

Breakfast:	Lush berry smoothie
Lunch:	Tuna lettuce cups
Dinner:	Spaghetti bolognaise minus the spaghetti

Saturday

Breakfast: Pesto scrambled eggs with mushrooms and tomatoes
Lunch: Tasty pecan chicken
Dinner: Roast lamb with broccolini

Sunday

Breakfast: Bubble and squeak
Lunch: Cauliflower salad with sardines
Dinner: Almond coated fish

12. Recipes to reverse Type 2 Diabetes

Breakfast recipes

Tomato Frittata - Serves 4

Ingredients

- 1 Tbsp olive oil
- 1 cup cauliflower flowerets
- 1 cup button mushrooms, sliced
- 6 eggs
- 1 Tbsp water
- 1/3 cup unsweetened soy or almond milk
- 1½ tsp dried oregano
- 1 tsp sweet (Hungarian) paprika
- 6 thin tomato slices
- ¼ cup grated parmesan cheese

Method

Combine the cauliflower, water and oil in a 10 inch pan or skillet. Cover and cook until softened slightly. Arrange mushrooms in the pan decoratively. Blend eggs, milk, oregano and paprika together well. Pour over cauliflower mixture. Cooked covered over medium heat until eggs are almost set.

Arrange tomato slices decoratively on top and sprinkle with cheese. Cover, and cook until eggs are completely set.

Cut into wedges and serve.

Strawberry delight smoothie - Serves 1

Ingredients

- ½ cup fresh strawberries
- 1 cup water or ¾ cup water and ¼ cup coconut milk
- 1 scoop vanilla Synd-X Slimming Whey Protein Powder

Method

Place all ingredients in blender and blend on high speed until smooth.

Omelet with cheese, asparagus and mushrooms - Serves 2

Ingredients

- 2 Tbsp olive oil
- 8 button mushrooms
- 1 Tbsp chopped parsley
- 2 tsp lemon juice
- 2 eggs, separated
- 1/3 cup thick natural yogurt
- 3 Tbsp grated parmesan cheese
- 6 asparagus spears, halved lengthwise
- Sea salt and pepper to taste

Method

Cook the mushrooms in olive oil in a saucepan over medium heat until softened (3-4 minutes). Add the lemon juice, parsley, salt and pepper. Take off the heat and keep warm.

Whisk the egg yolks and yogurt together. In a separate bowl, beat the egg whites to soft peaks and fold through the yolk mixture.

Brush a frying pan with a little olive oil and then pour in the omelet mixture. Cook until just set (4 minutes). Place the asparagus over half the omelet, and sprinkle the cheese over. Fold the omelet in half and cook for one more minute. Serve topped with the mushrooms.

Good Morning Squares - Serves 4

Ingredients

- 1 tsp baking powder
- 6 eggs
- ½ teaspoon cumin
- ¼ cup grated parmesan cheese
- ½ cup chopped red bell pepper
- ¾ cup grated Zucchini
- 2 Tbsp melted butter or olive oil
- 1 Tbsp chopped parsley
- ¼ cup chopped onion

Method

Preheat the oven to 350°F (180°C). Beat the eggs in a large bowl until well blended. Stir in baking powder well. Stir in remaining ingredients. Pour into greased 9 inch baking dish. Bake 30-35 minutes; until inserted knife comes out clean. Stand for at least 5 minutes before serving.

This breakfast is great made in advance, and taken with you when you have to eat on the run.

Peach and Nut Smoothie - Serves 1

Ingredients

- 1 medium peach, chopped
- 1 cup water
- 1 heaped tablespoon almond butter/paste
- 1 scoop Synd-X Slimming Whey Protein Powder

Method

Place all ingredients in a blender, blend on low speed first, then high speed until well blended. Scrape the sides of the blender with a spatula if needed. Add more water, or a pinch of stevia powder for your desired consistency and sweetness.

Mushroom Frittata - Serves 4

Ingredients

- 1 cup broccoli flowerets

- 1 cup sliced mushrooms

- ½ cup sliced red or green bell pepper

- ½ cup diced onion

- ½ cup flaked, drained tinned tuna

- 8 eggs

- ¼ cup water

- 1 tsp dried oregano

- 2 Tbsp grated parmesan cheese

Method

Grease a 10 inch omelet pan or skillet with olive oil. Make sure it has an ovenproof handle. Cook the broccoli, mushrooms, bell pepper and onion until just tender. Remove from heat; stir in tuna and set aside.

Beat the eggs, water and oregano together in a medium bowl. Pour over the vegetable mixture in pan and cook until the egg mixture sets at the edges; 5 to 8 minutes. Sprinkle with parmesan cheese and bake in a 375°F (190°C) preheated oven for 8 to 10 minutes. The top should be browned and set, with no liquid egg remaining.

This breakfast can be eaten fresh and hot, and you can save leftovers for lunch or for breakfast tomorrow.

Spinach Omelet - Serves 1

Ingredients

- 2 eggs
- ¼ cup chopped spinach
- 2 button mushrooms, sliced
- 1 Tbsp chopped onion
- 1 Tbsp soy or almond milk or water
- Sea salt and pepper to taste

Method

Beat the eggs. Combine all ingredients and pour into a frying pan. Cook without stirring for 2 minutes; then fold omelet in half.

Serve with fresh parsley.

Quick and Tasty Egg Breakfast

Ingredients

- Sliced tomatoes
- Sliced onion
- Pitted olives, sliced in half
- Sliced mushrooms

Method

In a frying pan, cook the above ingredients in olive oil, in a quantity that suits the number of people eating.

Once cooked, whisk some eggs together and pour into the frying pan to fill the holes. Sprinkle chopped Feta cheese on top. Sprinkle with salt, pepper and any other spices you like. Continue cooking until eggs have set. Serve.

Tropical Smoothie - Serves 1

Ingredients

- Pulp of 2 passionfruit
- 1 scoop Synd-X Slimming Whey Protein Powder
- ¼ cup coconut milk
- ¾ cup water

Method

Blend ingredients together and serve.

Salmon Omelet - Serves 1

Ingredients

- 3.5 ounce (100g) tin of salmon, drained
- 2 eggs
- 2 Tbsp Ricotta cheese
- 2 Tbsp olive oil
- 1 tsp chopped fresh dill
- ¼ cup finely diced green bell pepper
- Sea salt and black pepper to taste

Method

In a small bowl beat the eggs, Ricotta, dill and bell pepper; season with salt and pepper. Preheat the oven to 375°F (190°C). In a heavy, oven-proof frying pan heat the olive oil over medium heat. Pour the egg mixture into the pan and cook until the base is set.

Flake the canned salmon and arrange it over half of the omelet.

Place the frying pan in the oven and cook until the top of the omelet is set. Carefully fold the omelet in half and serve.

Low carb hash brown - Serves 1

Ingredients

- 1 cup grated zucchini; squeeze out excess moisture
- 2 eggs, beaten
- 1 Tbsp grated onion
- 1 clove garlic, minced (optional)
- ½ Tsp cumin
- 1 Tbsp olive oil
- Sea salt and black pepper to taste

Method

Combine all ingredients except olive oil together in a medium bowl; mash them well with your hand. Heat olive oil in a large frying pan over medium heat. Divide mixture into two hash browns and cook. When one side is cooked, flip over and cook the other side.

Lush Berry Smoothie - Serves 1

Ingredients

- ½ cup frozen berries of your choice
- ¼ cup Greek yogurt - unsweetened
- ¾ cup water
- ¼ cup canned coconut milk
- 2 Tbsp Synd-X Slimming Whey Protein Powder
- Stevia powder to taste – between 1 pinch and ¼ tsp

Method

Blend all ingredients in a blender then drink.

Pesto scrambled eggs with mushrooms and tomatoes - Serves 2

Ingredients

- 5 eggs
- ½ cup milk – either cow's milk or unsweetened non-dairy milk.
- 2 Tbsp butter or olive oil
- 1 tsp Pesto
- Sea salt and black pepper to taste
- 5 button mushrooms, chopped
- 2 small ripe Roma tomatoes cut in half

Method

Beat the eggs in a large bowl with a fork. Add the milk, Pesto, salt and pepper and continue beating. Heat the butter or olive oil in a large frying pan. Add the eggs and stir and scrape them around the pan frequently until they are cooked to your liking.

Place the eggs on serving plates.

Cook the mushrooms and tomatoes in the same frying pan until they are done to your liking. Serve.

Bubble and Squeak - Serves 1

Ingredients

- 1 cup of leftover cooked, mashed vegetables. Broccoli, cauliflower, green beans and carrots work well.
- 2 sun dried tomatoes, finely chopped
- 2 eggs, beaten with a fork
- Sea salt and black pepper to taste
- 1 Tbsp olive oil

Method

Mix all ingredients together and form into patties. Cook in olive oil in a frying pan until done to your liking.

Lunch recipes

Tuna Salad with Lime Mayonnaise - Serves 2

Ingredients

- 1 x 15 ounce (425g) can tuna in brine, olive oil or spring water
- ½ cup cooked green beans
- 1 small red onion, sliced
- 1/3 cup fresh cilantro or parsley, finely chopped
- 2 tsp capers
- 1/3 cup whole-egg mayonnaise
- 1 ½ Tbsp lime juice
- 1 tsp finely grated lime rind

Method

Combine the first five ingredients well in a bowl. Combine the last three ingredients and blend well. Place the salad on serving plates and spoon mayonnaise on top.

Chicken Avocado Salad - Serves 4

Ingredients

- 2 cooked chicken breasts, chopped
- 2 Roma tomatoes, sliced
- ½ cucumber, sliced
- 1 grated carrot
- 8 cos lettuce leaves, torn
- 1 avocado, sliced

- ¼ cup chopped fresh cilantro
- Olive oil and lime juice as dressing
- 1.8 ounces (50g) shaved parmesan cheese

Method

Toss all ingredients together in a bowl except the oil, lime juice and cheese. Drizzle olive oil and lime juice over the salad. Sprinkle with parmesan cheese and serve.

Tasty Lunchtime Rissoles - Makes approximately 8 rissoles

Ingredients

- 17.5 ounces (500g) lean ground beef
- 1 egg
- 1 onion, grated
- 2 Tbsp parsley, finely chopped
- 1 tsp turmeric
- 1 tsp sweet paprika
- 1 tsp cumin
- 2 cloves garlic, crushed (optional)
- Sea salt and black pepper to taste

Method

Preheat the oven to 350°F (180°C). In a large bowl mix all ingredients together thoroughly. Shape mixture into approximately 8 rissoles. Bake on a greased oven tray, covered with foil until cooked.

These are very handy taken to work with a salad.

Warm Bell Pepper and Zucchini with Sardines
- Serves 2

Ingredients

- 1 medium red bell pepper
- 1 medium zucchini
- 2 teaspoons olive oil
- 1 clove garlic, minced
- Fresh basil leaves to serve
- 2 x 3.5 ounce (100 gram) tins of sardines

Method

Slice bell pepper and Zucchini into strips. Cook in oil for 4-5 minutes, until lightly browned and slightly softened. Add garlic and cook for a further 3-5 minutes.

Serve with tinned sardines and torn fresh basil leaves.

Chicken and Grapefruit Salad - Serves 2

Ingredients

- 2 cups cooked chicken, diced
- 1 grapefruit, cut into bite sized pieces
- ½ Lebanese cucumber, sliced
- 1 avocado, sliced
- ½ small Spanish onion, sliced
- ¼ cup fresh cilantro, chopped
- ½ cup plain yogurt as dressing

Method

Combine all ingredients together and serve.

Salmon and Warm Vegetable Salad - Serves 4

Ingredients

- 2 red or green bell peppers
- 4 large button mushrooms, quartered
- 2 medium red onions cut into wedges
- 3 baby aubergines, sliced in half lengthways
- 3 medium squash, sliced lengthways
- Large handful of fresh basil leaves, torn into small pieces
- ¼ cup olive oil
- 14.5 ounce (415g) can pink or red salmon drained and flaked

HERB and GARLIC DRESSING

- 1 clove garlic, crushed
- 1/3 cup lemon juice
- 2 tablespoons olive oil

Method

Combine the dressing ingredients in a screw top jar and shake well.

Quarter the bell peppers; remove seeds and membranes. Brush the vegetables with oil and cook on an oiled grill or barbecue until tender and browned lightly. Remove the skin from the bell pepper. Combine the grilled vegetables with basil and toss in half the dressing. Place the salmon on top and drizzle with remaining dressing.

Lemony Chicken Salad - Serves 4

Ingredients

- 17.5 ounces (500g) cooked chicken, chopped
- 1 cup plain yogurt
- ½ red onion, chopped
- 4 radishes, sliced

- 2 Tbsp slivered almonds
- ½ Tsp grated lemon zest
- ½ cup torn basil leaves

Method

Mix all ingredients together in a bowl, ensuring they are well coated. Serve.

Chicken and Blueberry Salad - Serves 4

Ingredients

- 4 handfuls of arugula leaves or lettuce
- 2 cooked chicken breasts, chopped
- 1 cup blueberries
- 1 bunch cilantro, chopped
- 1 avocado, finely chopped
- 2 stalks celery, chopped
- 4 Tbsp slivered almonds
- Lemon juice and olive oil as dressing

Method

Combine all ingredients in a bowl; toss well and serve.

Sunflower Salad With Tuna - Serves 1

Ingredients

- 1 cup firmly packed grated carrot
- ½ cup thinly sliced celery
- 2 medium radishes, sliced
- 2 Tbsp sunflower seeds
- Lettuce leaves

- 1 Tbsp olive oil
- 1 Tbsp lemon juice
- 6.9 ounce (195g) tinned tuna

Method

Combine carrot, celery, radishes and sunflower seeds. Stir the oil and juice together. Arrange carrot mixture over lettuce leaves, pour dressing on top, and serve with tinned tuna.

Chicken and Artichoke Salad - Serves 3

Ingredients

- 14 ounces (400g) cooked chicken, cut into bite sized pieces
- 7 ounces (200g) artichokes in brine, drained and chopped
- 3 button mushrooms, chopped
- 4 radishes, chopped
- 3 sun-dried tomatoes, chopped
- Radicchio or other lettuce, torn into bite sized pieces
- 2 sticks celery, chopped
- Olive oil and lemon juice as dressing

Method

Mix salad ingredients together well. Pour olive oil and lemon juice on top and serve.

Salmon Salad - Serves 1

Ingredients

- 1 x 7 ounce (200g) can red or pink salmon
- 1 medium cooked beet, diced
- 1 stalk celery, sliced
- ½ cup button mushrooms, sliced

- Fresh cilantro leaves, chopped
- Olive oil and plain yogurt to dress

Method

Mix vegetables together. Add salmon and mix roughly. Drizzle with olive oil and dollop 2 tablespoons of plain yogurt on top.

Tuna Lettuce Cups - Serves 4

Ingredients

- 8 asparagus spears, chopped and cooked
- 4 large iceberg lettuce leaves
- 1 avocado, sliced
- ¼ cup slivered almonds
- 15 ounces (425g) tinned tuna
- 8 cherry tomatoes, halved
- ½ cup grated carrot
- ½ cup plain yogurt as dressing

Method

Combine asparagus, avocado, almonds, tuna, tomatoes and carrot well in a bowl. Scoop mixture into lettuce leaves and top with yogurt.

Tasty pecan chicken - Serves 4

Ingredients

1 cup ground pecans – grind them in a food processor or coffee grinder. You can use almond meal if you don't have one of these machines.

- ½ cup freshly grated parmesan cheese
- 4 chicken breast halves
- 2 Tbsp olive oil

- 1 Tbsp butter
- ½ Tsp ground cilantro
- 1 clove garlic, finely minced (optional)
- ¼ cup lemon juice
- Sea salt and black pepper to taste

Method

Pound the chicken breasts with a meat mallet to make them an even thickness.

Place the ground pecans, cheese, cilantro, garlic, salt and pepper in a shallow bowl. Put the lemon juice into another shallow bowl.

Dip both sides of the chicken breasts in lemon juice then coat in pecan mixture. Heat the olive oil and butter in a large frying pan on medium heat. Cook the chicken until golden brown; approximately 3 to 5 minutes on each side.

Serve with a salad or cooked vegetables.

Cauliflower salad with Sardines - Serves 2

Ingredients

- ¼ head of cauliflower, cooked, well drained and chopped
- 2 Tbsp olive or macadamia nut oil
- 2 Tbsp lime juice
- ¼ cup chopped red bell pepper
- 2 stalks celery, chopped
- ¼ cup finely chopped scallions
- ¼ cup finely chopped fresh parsley
- 2 x 3.5 ounce (100 gram) tins of sardines

Method

Combine all ingredients except oil and lime juice. Whisk oil and juice together in a bowl until well combined. Pour over salad and serve.

Dinner recipes

Baked Chicken Breasts With Lemon and Feta

- Serves 4

Ingredients

- 2 Tbsp olive oil
- 1 Tbsp lemon juice
- 21 ounces (600 grams) chicken breast fillets
- ¼ cup fresh basil leaves
- 2 Tbsp grated lemon zest
- 4.2 ounces (120 grams) Feta cheese, crumbled

Method

Preheat the oven to 400°F (200°C). Place the oil and lemon juice in a baking dish, add the chicken and coat it well. Leave for 5 minutes. Add the basil and lemon zest, and sprinkle the Feta on top.

Bake for 30 minutes or until cooked through. Serve with a salad or steamed vegetables.

Middle Eastern Fish - Serves 4

Ingredients

- Fish fillets of your choice to serve 4
- 1 fluid ounce (30 mL) lemon juice
- 1 Tbsp olive oil
- Sea salt and black pepper to taste
- 2 Tbsp chopped fresh dill
- 1 large onion, sliced finely
- 4.4 ounces (125g) tahini (sesame paste)
- 1 clove garlic, minced (optional)
- Juice of 3 lemons

Method

Preheat the oven to 400°F (200°Celsius). Mix the tahini with 30 mL (1 oz.) lemon juice, garlic, sea salt and pepper. Add enough water so that it becomes a thick sauce. Sprinkle the fish with a little sea salt and the juice from 3 lemons. Let it stand for 30 minutes. Drain the fish, place the sliced onion on top and brush with olive oil.

Bake the fish for 20 minutes. Pour the tahini sauce on top and continue baking until cooked; when the fish flakes easily.

Sprinkle the fresh dill over the fish and serve with salad or steamed vegetables.

Herb Coated Veal - Serves 8

Ingredients

- 2.2 pounds (1kg) veal loin
- 1 Tbsp olive oil
- Sea salt and black pepper to taste
- 1 ½ Tbsp Dijon mustard
- 1 Tbsp lemon juice
- 1 clove garlic, crushed (optional)
- 2 Tbsp parsley, finely chopped

Method

Preheat the oven to 400°F (200°C). Rub the oil over the veal and top with salt and pepper. Sear the veal for 4 minutes each side on a hot frying pan. Spread the lemon juice and mustard over the veal. Roast the veal in the oven until cooked. Combine the crushed garlic and parsley; rub over the veal once it has cooled slightly; serve warm with a salad or cooked vegetables.

Chicken Soup - Serves 4

Ingredients

- 1 Tbsp olive oil
- 2 red bell peppers, finely chopped

- 1 stalk celery, sliced
- 1 leek, finely sliced
- 4 garlic cloves, finely chopped
- 2 zucchini, chopped
- 1 carrot, chopped
- 7 cups water or chicken stock
- 17.6 ounces (500 grams) chicken breasts, chopped finely
- ½ Tsp dried thyme
- 2 bay leaves
- Sea salt and black pepper to taste

Method

Heat olive oil in large saucepan over medium heat. Add chicken, bell pepper, celery and leek; cook for approximately 8 minutes. Add a small amount of water if needed. Add garlic and stir in water or stock, thyme and bay leaves.

Bring to boil, reduce heat to simmer and cook covered for 25 minutes. Add salt, pepper and zucchini; cook a further 15 minutes, until zucchini is tender. Add more water if required. Serve and enjoy.

Salmon Steaks with Fennel - Serves 4

Ingredients

- 4 salmon steaks
- 1 lemon, juiced
- 3 Tbsp fresh fennel fronds, chopped
- 1 tsp dried fennel seeds
- Sea salt and black pepper to taste
- 1 Tbsp olive oil

Method

Mix together in a bowl the fennel fronds and seeds, lemon juice and olive oil. Pour this mixture over the salmon, sprinkle with salt and pepper, and refrigerate for 2 hours. Fry, grill or barbecue the salmon and serve with a salad or steamed vegetables.

Stir-Fried Aubergine and Tomatoes with Lamb Chops - Serves 3

Ingredients

- 6 lean lamb chops, visible fat removed
- 1 Tbsp olive oil
- ½ large or 1 small aubergine, peeled and diced
- 1 stalk celery, sliced
- 1 onion, diced
- 2 small squash, diced
- 1 large or 2 small well ripened tomatoes, chopped
- 1 Tbsp balsamic vinegar
- 1 tsp dried cilantro or cumin
- Sea salt and black pepper to taste
- ½ cup chopped parsley

Method

Grill lamb chops until cooked to your liking. Keep warm.

Heat olive oil in wok or large frying pan. Cook aubergine, celery, onion and squash on medium heat for 7-10 minutes. Add remaining ingredients, cover and simmer for 20 minutes; adding some water if needed. Serve over 2 lamb chops for each person.

Grilled Salmon with Avocado Salsa - Serves 4

Ingredients

- 4 salmon fillets
- 2 medium avocados, sliced
- 1 medium red onion, sliced
- ¼ red bell pepper, diced finely
- 2 Tbsp capers, drained
- Large handful arugula
- LIME DRESSING
- 2 Tbsp lime juice
- 1/3 cup olive oil
- Sea salt and black pepper

Method

Cook salmon on an oiled grill or frying pan for approximately 4 minutes each side. Combine the avocado, onion, bell pepper, capers, arugula and dill in a medium bowl.

Combine the dressing ingredients in a screw top jar and shake well. Serve the salmon with salsa on top; drizzled with lime dressing.

Veal Cutlets - Serves 4

Ingredients

- 1 lemon
- 8 veal cutlets
- 1 Tbsp fresh thyme or sage leaves
- 2 cloves garlic, crushed
- ¼ cup olive oil
- Sea salt and pepper to taste

Method

Grate the rind of the lemon thinly and place in a large bowl. Add the remaining ingredients except the salt and pepper. Coat the cutlets well, cover and refrigerate overnight.

Sprinkle salt and pepper over the cutlets and cook on an oiled grill or barbecue until browned on both sides. Serve with fresh salad vegetables.

Chicken With Olives - Serves 2

Ingredients

- 2 small chicken breasts
- 2 Tbsp olive oil
- 1 onion, sliced
- 2 cloves garlic, sliced
- 4 medium button squash, quartered
- 14 ounce (400g) tin diced tomatoes
- 1 Tbsp dried oregano
- 1 tsp sweet paprika
- ¼ cup black olives
- 1 Tbsp capers

Method

Preheat oven to 400°F (200°C). Cook chicken breasts in 1 tablespoon of oil in a frying pan over high heat. Remove from heat when browned. Combine remaining ingredients together in a bowl. Transfer into a baking dish and top with chicken breasts.

Cover with foil and bake for 20 minutes. Remove foil and bake a further 10 minutes. Serve with a salad.

Gingery Chicken - Serves 2

Ingredients

- 12 ounces (350g) chicken breast, sliced
- 2 cloves garlic, crushed (optional)

- 1 tsp grated fresh ginger root
- Juice of ½ lemon
- 1 Tbsp olive oil
- ½ cup water
- 1 carrot, sliced into matchsticks
- 2 cups shredded Chinese cabbage
- ¼ cup raw cashew pieces
- 1 Tbsp tamari (wheat free soy sauce)

Method

Cook the chicken, garlic and ginger root in the oil and lemon in a wok or frying pan until the chicken is golden. Add the remaining ingredients and cook until the carrot has softened slightly. Serve.

Almond Coated Fish - Serves 2

Ingredients

- 2 fish fillets of your choice
- ½ cup slivered almonds
- 1 clove garlic, minced
- Hungarian (sweet) paprika to taste
- 1 Tbsp olive oil

Method

Rub the fish with olive oil and garlic. Coat with slivered almonds and paprika. Fry in pan until cooked. Serve with a salad or cooked vegetables.

Pork Meatball Soup - Serves 4

Ingredients

- 8 cups water or vegetable stock
- 6 large button mushrooms, chopped
- 1 bunch bok choy, chopped
- 1 leek, sliced finely

MEATBALLS

- 14 ounces (400g) minced pork
- ½ bunch English spinach, finely chopped
- 2 cloves garlic, minced (optional)
- 1 tsp tamari
- 1 tsp ground cumin

Method

Mix meatball ingredients together to form approximately 20-25 meatballs.

Bring stock to the boil, reduce to simmer and gently add meatballs, mushrooms and leek. Cook covered for approximately 30 minutes. Add bok choy and cook a further 5 minutes. Serve.

Spaghetti Bolognaise minus the Spaghetti

Cook your usual spaghetti bolognaise, (choose a tomato sauce without added sugar, or make your own), and instead of having it with spaghetti, pour it over your favorite cooked vegetables (e.g. Broccoli, cauliflower, green beans, zucchini, mushrooms, etc.)

Roast Lamb with Broccolini - Serves 2

Ingredients

- 7 ounces (200g) lamb loin (or lamb fillet or lamb backstraps)
- 2 Tbsp olive oil
- 1 lemon, unpeeled and cut into slices
- 1 Tbsp balsamic vinegar
- 1 bunch broccolini, cut in half
- 1 handful snow peas, trimmed

Method

Preheat the oven to 400°F (200°C). Place the lamb into a greased oven-proof dish. Arrange the lemon slices over the lamb and drizzle half the olive oil and all of the balsamic vinegar over it. Roast the lamb in the oven for 15 minutes.

Toss the broccolini and snow peas in the remaining olive oil, sprinkle with sea salt and pepper if desired. Add the vegetables to the lamb and continue roasting for another 15 minutes or longer, depending on how you like your lamb.

Cover the lamb with foil and let it rest for 5 minutes before slicing it. Serve with a green salad.

Vegetarian Recipes

Chickpea and Sesame Salad - Serves 2

Ingredients

- 1 can of chickpeas, rinsed and drained
- ½ cup dry roasted sesame seeds*
- ½ cup cooked green beans, chopped
- ½ bunch fresh cilantro
- ½ cup fresh mint
- 2 tomatoes
- 1 carrot
- 2 sticks celery
- 1 small bunch arugula
- ½ cup finely chopped parsley
- ½ cup finely cubed Feta cheese
- ½ red onion

DRESSING INGREDIENTS

- Add the following ingredient to your regular mayonnaise: juice of ½ a lime
- 1 tsp cumin powder
- 1 tsp cumin seeds

Method

Cut the carrot and celery into small cubes. Finely chop the onion, herbs and tomatoes.

Mix all together in a salad bowl. Add all remaining ingredients and mix through dressing. Serve.

* To dry roast place seeds into a skillet and brown over medium heat, stirring often. Be careful not to burn them.

Dahl Palak (Spinach with Split Peas) - Serves 2

Ingredients

- 1 cup Feta cheese cut into small cubes
- ½ cup split peas
- 1 ½ cups water
- ½ Tsp turmeric
- ½ Tsp salt
- 2 bunches English spinach
- 3 tsp ghee or organic coconut oil
- 2 cloves garlic, crushed (optional)
- 1 Tbsp garam masala
- 1 Tbsp lemon juice
- 1 Tbsp lime juice
- 1 Tbsp grated fresh ginger root
- ½ bunch fresh cilantro, finely chopped for garnish

Method

Soak split peas in a saucepan with 1 ½ cups of water for one hour. Add the turmeric and salt to peas and boil for 10 minutes. Wash fresh spinach and chop finely; cook for 5 minutes in 2 tablespoons of salted water. Drain all liquid.

Add spinach to split peas and cook slowly until most of the liquid is absorbed and the peas are cooked.

Heat ghee or coconut oil in a skillet. Add the ginger root and crushed garlic. Cook until the garlic is golden brown. Add garam masala. Add to saucepan with peas and spinach. Add lemon and lime juice; mix well. Place mixture on serving plates.

Mix the cubed Feta with fresh cilantro. Arrange over pea and spinach mixture on serving plates. Serve with a fresh salad.

Lentil Burgers - Serves 4

Ingredients

- 2 cups cooked brown lentils
- 2 cups cooked chickpeas
- 1 carrot, grated
- ½ brown onion, grated
- 2 Tbsp finely chopped parsley
- ½ cup finely chopped chives
- 1 cup finely chopped cilantro
- 1 Tbsp hot Indian curry paste
- 2 tsp cumin
- 1 Tbsp tomato puree
- 1 beaten egg
- Sea salt and black pepper to taste
- Blanched flaked almonds for coating
- Organic coconut oil for cooking

Method

Mash the chickpeas and lentils together by hand or with a food processor. Add all other ingredients together except the egg, almonds and oil. Mix thoroughly together.

Add beaten egg and mix well. Heat oil in pan and put flaked almonds in a bowl – crush them with your fingers first.

Roll the lentil mixture into patties and coat them in almonds. Fry them in coconut oil until browned. Serve with a fresh salad or spicy tomato salsa.

Spinach and Chickpeas - Serves 3

Ingredients

- 2 fresh bunches of spinach
- 1 cup cooked chickpeas
- 2 tsp curry powder
- 1 clove garlic, crushed (optional)
- 1 brown onion, chopped
- 1 cup water
- 2 Tbsp olive oil
- 1 tsp cumin
- Juice of ¼ fresh lemon or ½ fresh lime
- ½ bunch fresh cilantro, chopped
- ½ cup dry roasted sesame seeds
- ¼ cup walnuts

Method

Cook spinach in 3 tablespoons of water then drain well. Cook onion in olive oil for 3 minutes. Add the garlic to the pan. Add the water, curry powder, spices, lemon or lime juice and chopped cilantro. Add the spinach and chickpeas to the mixture.

Cook stirring for 2 minutes, then simmer covered for 5 minutes. Serve. Sprinkle sesame seeds and walnuts on top.

Bean soup - Serves 4

You can buy a variety of tinned beans in all supermarkets. Just remember to read the labels and avoid those that contain added sugar. If you want to really get your hands dirty you can soak dried beans in water overnight to use in this recipe.

Ingredients

- 1 cup canned or pre-soaked chickpeas
- 1 cup canned or pre-soaked kidney beans
- 1 cup canned or pre-soaked Lima beans
- 1 cup canned or pre-soaked lentils
- 3 Tbsp olive oil
- 2 carrots
- 3 celery sticks
- 1 large brown onion
- 1 clove garlic, crushed
- 1 cup fresh basil, chopped
- ¼ Tsp chili powder
- 1 Tsp cumin
- 1 sprig rosemary – remove stalk
- ½ cup fresh peas
- 2 Tbsp tamari
- 1 Tbsp miso paste (optional)
- 2 cups V8 vegetable juice
- 4 cups water
- ½ cup parsley, finely chopped
- Sea salt and black pepper to taste
- 1 turnip
- 1 vegetable stock cube
- 2 bay leaves
- ½ cup pine nuts – dry roasted and lightly crushed

Method

In a frying pan heat the oil and add finely chopped onion. Cook for 3 minutes then add crushed garlic. Cook for 2 minutes.

Transfer onion mixture into a large soup pot. Chop carrots, celery and turnip into small cubes; add to pot. Add V8 juice, chili, cumin, rosemary, peas, tamari, miso, stock cube, salt, pepper and water. Stir. Cook covered on medium to low heat for 5 minutes, then add lentils. Cook covered slowly for another 20 minutes, and then add all beans, bay leaves and fresh basil.

Add a little of the fresh parsley and save the rest for a garnish. Cook soup gently until the vegetables and beans are soft. Mix the crushed pine nuts with the chopped parsley.

Place soup into serving bowls and sprinkle with pine nut and parsley combination.

4 Bean Salad - Serves 3

Ingredients

- 1 can 4 bean mix, rinsed and drained
- 1 cup green peas, cooked
- 1 cup finely chopped spinach
- 1 small red onion, finely chopped
- 1 cup chopped walnuts
- ½ cup pepitas
- 2 tomatoes, chopped finely
- 2 sticks celery, finely chopped
- 3 sun dried tomatoes, finely chopped
- ½ cup olives
- ½ bunch fresh basil, finely chopped
- 2 Tbsp finely chopped mint leaves
- 1 carrot, finely chopped
- 1 cup grated parmesan cheese
- ½ cup finely chopped parsley

Method

In a salad bowl place the beans, peas, spinach, onion, tomatoes, celery, sun dried tomatoes, olives, basil, mint and carrot. Place the pepitas and walnuts in a skillet and dry roast them until golden brown; be careful not to burn them. Let them cool and add to the salad.

Place salad onto serving bowls and garnish with grated parmesan and parsley.

For a dressing add a little chili powder, coconut cream and fresh lime juice to your regular mayonnaise.

Maintenance: how to keep Diabetes at bay

Many of the dietary changes you make on this Diabetes eating plan will need to become permanent habits. If you revert back to your old habits, you will surely gain weight again and your blood sugar will rise.

The most important principle to remember is to *eat protein at each meal.* This can be lean meat, fish, chicken, eggs or a whey based protein powder. This will ensure that your blood sugar level remains stable throughout the day; helping to prevent cravings, and excessive hunger. It is always important to include beneficial fats in your diet also, such as olive oil, avocados, oily fish and nuts and seeds.

Most people can reintroduce grains and starchy vegetables back into their diet, in small quantities. They must be whole grain, low glycemic index carbohydrates such as rye bread, sweet potatoes and whole grain pasta. You can also include more legumes in your diet if you wish. How much of these foods you will be able to eat depends on how much exercise you do, your age and how long you have been a diabetic. Whenever you make dietary changes please keep a close eye on your blood sugar level and weight; that way you will know the impact these changes are having.

If you find that your weight is creeping up again and your blood sugar is rising, reduce your carbohydrate intake again, and these should come down.

Type 1 Diabetes in more detail

Type 1 Diabetes is an autoimmune disease whereby the immune system attacks and destroys the insulin producing cells in the pancreas. Therefore the pancreas is no longer able to produce sufficient insulin and blood sugar rises because it is not able to enter the cells. There are many different kinds of autoimmune diseases, for example rheumatoid arthritis, multiple sclerosis, lupus and Hashimoto's thyroiditis; in all cases the immune system mistakenly identifies part of the body as a foreign invader and produces antibodies to attack it. Type 1 Diabetes usually develops in childhood; it is also known as juvenile onset Diabetes or insulin dependant Diabetes mellitus. It is far less common than Type 2 Diabetes; it makes up only ten to 15 percent of all cases of Diabetes. It is more common in Caucasians than other racial groups.

Worldwide there has been a three to ten-fold increase in the incidence of type 1 Diabetes in the last 40 years. Genetic factors are commonly blamed for the development of this disease, but the truth is they only play a small part in type 1 Diabetes. Dietary and environmental factors are much more important in the causation of this disease. When one identical twin has type 1 Diabetes, the other twin only develops the disease in 23 to 38 percent of cases.[35,36] Type 1 Diabetes is very rare among Polynesians but the rate increases more than seven-fold when Polynesians migrate to New Zealand. This just shows how important environmental and dietary factors are in this disease.

Most of the risk factors associated with type 1 Diabetes are related to immune system dysfunction.

Risk factors for developing type 1 Diabetes

• 	Abnormalities of the gut immune system.

• Approximately 70 to 80 percent of the immune cells in your body live in your digestive tract. The immune cells here survey the food molecules and microbes that you ingest and react appropriately to protect your body against allergies and infections. In type 1 Diabetes the gut immune system malfunctions and ultimately leads to the production of antibodies that attack and destroy the beta cells of the pancreas.

A number of factors can contribute to this immune dysfunction, including not being breast fed, or being breast fed for less than six months, early weaning (before six months) and being born through caesarian section, rather than a natural birth. Children who develop type 1 Diabetes usually have poor protein digestion, this means complete proteins are able to enter the bloodstream undigested and stimulate the formation of antibodies against them. This is usually a forerunner to autoimmune disease.

• Intolerance to dairy products and/or gluten.

• Components of cow's milk protein (casein) and gluten are similar to proteins on the beta cells of the pancreas. This means a faulty immune system can cross-react and start forming antibodies against the beta cells if a food intolerance exists. Early introduction of cow's milk and gluten (before the age of 12 months) increases the risk of type 1 Diabetes. Children with gluten intolerance (coeliac disease) are three times more likely to be diagnosed with type 1 Diabetes.37

• Viral infections of the gastrointestinal tract.

• Infection with either enteroviruses or rotaviruses is very common in children and generally produces diarrhea. All of these viruses replicate in the digestive tract and stimulate the immune system there. These viruses can also infect the beta cells of the pancreas, which stimulates white blood cells to attack and destroy these cells, in an effort to kill the virus.

Viral gastrointestinal infections also increase the permeability of the intestinal tract, making it leaky. Leaky gut syndrome increases the absorption of incompletely digested proteins and toxins into the bloodstream, where they stress the immune system.

• Vitamin D deficiency. Studies have shown that people newly diagnosed with type 1 Diabetes have much lower blood levels of vitamin D than healthy people. Vitamin D supplementation during pregnancy and early childhood does reduce the risk of a child developing type 1 Diabetes. A study conducted in Finland recruited more than 12,000 pregnant women who were due to give birth in 1966. Their children were monitored until 1997. The results of this study showed that children who regularly took vitamin D supplements had an 80 percent reduced risk of developing type 1 Diabetes. The children who had a vitamin D deficiency were actually 300 percent more likely to develop type 1 Diabetes![38]

The vitamin D used in this study was primarily from cod liver oil supplements. Vitamin D is also available as a supplement on its own, and it is found in egg yolks, fish and some dairy products. Your body also makes vitamin D when your skin is exposed to sunlight.

• Omega 3 fatty acid deficiency.

Omega 3 fats have a powerful anti inflammatory effect in the body and they help to keep cell membranes healthy, allowing proper cell function. These fats improve the function of the immune cells in the digestive tract. Children who are deficient in omega 3 fatty acids have higher rates of type 1 Diabetes.

• Nitrates and nitrosamines.

These compounds are strongly linked to the development of type 1 Diabetes. Nitrates are created by agricultural runoff from fertilizers, therefore can make their way into the water supply. The increasing use of nitrogen fertilizers has increased the concentration of nitrates in ground water worldwide. Nitrates are also found in smoked or cured meats such as bacon, ham, hotdogs and jerky, to prevent them from going off. Nitrates are converted into nitrosamines in the stomach and both of these compounds are known to cause Diabetes in animals. Everybody should avoid eating nitrate containing meat, especially children.

Diet guidelines for Type 1 Diabetics

People with type 1 Diabetes should not follow the eating plan in this book unless they have the supervision of their doctor or other health care practitioner. If you have type 1 Diabetes, you should also keep your intake of carbohydrates low and avoid becoming overweight, because this will help to keep your blood sugar level stable. Just like people with Syndrome X have become resistant to the hormone insulin, so too people with type 1 Diabetes can become resistant to the insulin they inject. If you are a type 1 diabetic with insulin resistance you are at high risk of cardiovascular disease and other complications of Diabetes.

If you follow a high carbohydrate diet and gain weight you will need to use more insulin; over time the insulin will make you gain even more weight, especially around your abdomen and make it harder for you to keep your blood sugar down. The more your blood sugar rises, the more insulin you will need to use. The less carbohydrate you eat, the less insulin you need to use.

Type 1 diabetics often develop the complications of Diabetes earlier in life; therefore they experience a much more severe version of them. This makes sense since the longer you have Diabetes; the more prone you are to its complications. If you have been a diabetic since childhood you are obviously at more risk than if you developed it in your forties.

In addition to following a low carbohydrate eating plan, most type 1 diabetics are best off avoiding dairy products and gluten. This can help with blood sugar control and reduces the risk of further immune system problems. Ensuring you have adequate vitamin D and omega 3 essential fatty acids is also essential if you have type 1 Diabetes.

The majority of the recommendations in this book are equally applicable to both type 1 and type 2 diabetics. However, if you are a type 1 diabetic please seek your doctor's advice before following them.

Conclusion

High blood sugar is a global killer; according to research published in *The Lancet* it is among the world's top five killers. High blood sugar starts causing health problems as soon as it becomes higher than normal; you don't even have to be a diabetic to fall into that category. Of all the diabetic complications discussed in this book it is cardiovascular disease that kills the majority of people. So much attention is focused on cholesterol levels, but high blood sugar may be even more relevant in promoting heart attacks and strokes.

Hopefully we have educated you and answered your questions about Diabetes. The more informed you are about your health condition, the more power you have to do something about it. With the right diet and lifestyle choices you won't just be able to manage Type 2 Diabetes, you can actually reverse it.

So many diabetics spend a great deal of their life frustrated with not being able to lose weight. After reading this book it should be clear to you that it is not the quantity of fat in your diet that keeps you overweight, it is the carbohydrate. To keep your blood sugar and weight in the healthy range for the rest of your life you need to keep active, eat plenty of vegetables and most importantly watch your carbohydrate intake. The global fondness for sugar and flour containing foods is responsible for much of the obesity and Type 2 Diabetes in the world today.

Please remain under the care of your own doctor and inform them of any major dietary changes you wish to make. We are also available to help you; please feel free to contact us via the following methods:

In The United States of America

Phone 623 334 3232
Postal mail: PO Box 5070 Glendale AZ 85312-5070 USA

In Australia

Phone (02) 4655 8855
Postal mail – PO Box 689 Camden NSW 2570 Australia

Email –   contact@weightcontroldoctor.com
Internet – www.liverdoctor.com
                www.weightcontroldoctor.com

Glossary

- **Albuminuria -** High levels of a protein called albumin in the urine. May indicate kidney disease.

- **Beta cells -** The cells in the pancreas that are responsible for insulin production.

- **Creatinine -** A waste product removed by the kidneys. The amount of creatinine in blood and urine can reveal whether the kidneys are functioning properly.

- **Fructosamine -** A protein found in the blood that has glucose bound to it. Similar to glycosylated hemoglobin but indicates blood sugar level over the previous two to three weeks.

- **Gestational -** Refers to pregnancy, from the time of conception to delivery.

- **Glomerulus -** A tiny bunch of blood vessels that forms part of the filtering system of the kidneys.

- **Glucagon -** A hormone produced in the pancreas that raises blood glucose levels.

- **Glucose -** The type of sugar found in the blood. It is the body's main source of fuel.

- **Glucose tolerance test -** A test used to diagnose Diabetes or insulin resistance (Syndrome X). It involves drinking a 75 gram dose of glucose (after an overnight fast), followed by a series of blood tests, usually lasting two hours or more.

- **Glycosylated hemoglobin -** Hemoglobin with glucose and other sugars chemically attached to it. Hemoglobin A1c is a specific component of glycosylated hemoglobin. Also called glycated hemoglobin.

- **Hyperglycemia -** High blood glucose levels.

- **Hypoglycemia -** Low blood glucose levels. This can occur if a person with Diabetes has not eaten enough food, has exercised without eating enough food prior or has injected too much insulin. Symptoms of Hypoglycemia can include feeling shaky, dizzy, sweaty, having a headache and feeling very hungry.

- **Impaired Glucose Tolerance -** A blood glucose level that is higher than normal but not high enough to be diagnosed as diabetic. People with impaired glucose tolerance have Syndrome X and the majority of them go on to develop Type 2 Diabetes unless they make dietary changes.

- **Insulin -** A hormone produced by beta cells in the pancreas that lowers blood glucose.

- **Insulin Resistance -** Also known as Syndrome X. This condition occurs when the pancreas manufactures plenty of insulin but the body's cells no longer respond to it properly. This is due to obesity and other factors. Insulin resistance is a forerunner to Type 2 Diabetes.

- **Ketoacidosis -** Diabetic ketoacidosis is severe high blood sugar that requires immediate treatment. Blood sugar becomes extremely high but the sugar cannot get inside cells and be used for energy, therefore the body burns fat stores for energy and this results in the production of large numbers of ketone bodies (acids) in the body.

- **Ketone Bodies (Ketones) -** Substances produced in the body as a result of the breakdown of fat. If they reach high levels in diabetics they can be harmful.

- **Ketosis -** This occurs when the body uses its fat stores for energy and as a result, ketone bodies are produced. This is a normal, not harmful metabolic state in healthy individuals that results in weight loss.

- **Macrovascular -** Refers to the large blood vessels in the body.

- **Microvascular -** Refers to the tiny blood vessels in the body.

- **Nephropathy -** Kidney disease.

- **Neuropathy -** Disease of the nerves.

- **Pancreas -** An organ that sits behind the lower part of the stomach and produces the hormone insulin. The pancreas also produces some other hormones, including glucagon and enzymes required for the digestion of food.

- **Prandial -** Refers to meals. Pre-prandial means before meals; post-prandial means after meals.

- **Proteinuria -** The presence of protein in the urine. This may indicate kidney disease.

- **Renal -** Refers to the kidneys.

- **Retinopathy -** A disease of the tiny blood vessels in the retina of the eyes. It is a common complication of Diabetes and can lead to impaired vision and blindness.

References

1. World Diabetes Foundation

2. (www.smh.com.au World Diabetes Bill Skyrockets December 6, 2006

3. The IDF consensus worldwide definition of the metabolic syndrome. International Diabetes Federation

4. Michael T Murray ND, Michael R Lyon, MD How to Prevent and Treat Diabetes with Natural Medicine. Riverhead Books, New York 2003.

5. Rivellese AA, De Natale C, Lilli S. Type of dietary fat and insulin resistance. Ann NY Acad Sci. 2002;967:329-335.

6. Gloyn AL, McCarthy MI. The genetics of Type 2 Diabetes. Best Pract Res Clin Endocrinol Metab. 2001;15:293-308.

7. Diabetes poised to wipe out Aborigines. The Australian. Stephen Lunn, November 13, 2006-12-30

8. Bakris GL. Preserving renal function in adults with hypertension and Diabetes: a consensus approach. National Kidney Foundation Hypertension and Diabetes Executive Committees Working Group. Am J Kidney Dis. 2000;36(3):646-661.

9. Canadian Diabetes Association

10. Bjornholt JV, Erikssen G, Aaser E, Sandvik L, Nitter-Hauge S, Jervell J, Erikssen J, Thaulow E. Fasting blood glucose: an underestimated risk factor for cardiovascular death: results: results from a 22-year follow-up of healthy nondiabetic men. Diabetes Care 1999;22(1):45-49.

11. Coutinho M, Gersetin HC, Wang Y, Yusuf S. The relationship between glucose and incident cardiovascular events: a metaregression analysis of published data from 20 studies of 95,783 individuals followed for 12.4 years. Diabetes Care 22(2):233-240.

12. Diabetes Care 2006;29.2688-93

13. Avandia may increase risk of hip and other fractures www.Diabetesincontrol.com

14. Tappy, L. Thermic effect of food and sympathetic nervous system activity in humans. Reproduction Nutrition Development 1996;36:391-397.

15. Mikkelsen, PB., Toubro, S., Astrup, A. Effect of fat-reduced diets on 24 h energy expenditure: comparisons between animal protein, vegetable protein, and carbohydrate. American Journal of Clinical Nutrition 2000; 72:1135-1141.

16. McAuley, KA., Smith, KJ., Taylor, RW., McLay, RT., Williams, SM., Mann, JI. Long-term effects of popular dietary approaches on weight loss and features of insulin resistance. International Journal of Obesity 2006; 30:342-349.

17. Diabetes Care, Vol 6, Issue 4 328-333, 1983

18. The Diabetes Control and Complications Trial Research Group: The effect of intensive treatment of Diabetes on the development and progression of long-term complications in insulin-dependant Diabetes mellitus. N Engl Med 1993, 329:977-986

19. The Lancet 1964; 2(7349):6-8

20. Surender K Arora and Samy I McFarlane The case for low carbohydrate diets in Diabetes management Nutrition and Metabolism 2005, 2:16

21. Jorgen Vesti Nielsen, Per Westerlund and Per Bygren A low carbohydrate diet may prevent end-stage renal failure in Type 2 Diabetes. A case report. Nutrition and Metabolism 2006, 3:23

22. The New England Journal of Medicine February 7, 2002;346:393-403

23. Jiang R, Manson JE, Stampfer MJ, et al. Nut and peanut butter consumption and risk of Type 2 Diabetes in women. JAMA 2002;288(20):2554-2560

24. Journal of Nutrition 136:2987-2992, 2006

25. American Chemical Society's Journal of Agricultural and Food Chemistry, Jan 5, 2007

26. Eduardo Salazar-Martinez MD, PhD, Walter C Willett MD et al. Coffee consumption and risk for Type 2 Diabetes mellitus Annuals of Internal Medicine. 6 January 2004 | Volume 140 Issue 1 | Pages 1-8

27. - Gymnema Sylvestre - Use of Gymnema Sylvestre Leaf Extract in the control of blood glucose in insulin-dependent diabetes mellitus, Shanmugasundaram. G et al. Dept. Biochemistry, University of Madras, Madras 600-113, Elsevier Scientific Publishers Ireland 1990 Studies on the Hypoglycemic Action of Gymnema Sylvestre, Dept. Biochemistry, University of Madras 600 042, Arogya -J. Health Sci., 1981, VII, 38-60. Antidiabetic Effect of a leaf extract from Gymnema Sylvestre in non-insulin dependent diabetes mellitus patients, K. Baskaran et al. Journal of Ethnopharmacology, 30(1990) 295-305, Elsevier Scientific Publishers Ireland Ltd.

27A. - Momordica charantia (Bitter Melon)

27B. - Chromium - Kaats g et al. Effects of chromium picolinate on body composition. A randomized double-masked, placebo-controlled study. Current Therap. Research (1996) 57(10):747-765 Anderson RA et al. Elevated intakes of supplemental chromium improve glucose and insulin variables in individuals with type II diabetes. Diabetes (1997);46:1786-91 Cunningham JJ. Micronutrients as nutraceutical interventions in diabetes mellitus. J. Am Coll Nutr. 1998;17(1):7-10

28. - Lipoic Acid - Sachse G & Willms B. Efficiency of thioctic acid (lipoic acid) in the therapy of peripheral diabetic neuropathy. Hormone & Metabolic Research (Supplement). 9:105, 1980 Wagh SS et al. Mode of action of lipoic acid in diabetes. Journal of Bioscience. 11:59-74, 1987. Chromium Picolinate Liu, V. J., Chromium & Insulin in young subjects with normal glucose tolerance. Am. J. Clin. Nutr. 25(4) 1982, pp. 661-667 Jacob S. et al. Enhancement of glucose disposal in patients with type 2 diabetes by alpha-lipoic acid. Arzneim - Rorsch Drug Res. 1995;45(2):872-874 Jacob S. et al. The antioxidant alpha-lipoic acid enhances insulin-stimulated glucose metabolism

in insulin-resistant rat skeletal muscle. Diabetes. 1996;45:1024-1029 Jacobs et al. Enhancement of glucose disposal in patients with type 11 diabetes by alpha-lipoic acid. Arzneimittel-Forschung (1993) 45:87274 Strodter D et al. The influence of lipoic acid (thioctic acid) on metabolism and function of the diabetic heart. Diabetic Res. Clin. Prac. (1995) 29(1):19-26 Packer L et al. Neuro protection by the metabolic antioxidant alpha lipoic acid. Free Radical Biol. Med. (1997) 22(1-2): 359-78 Khamaisis M: Lipoic acid reduces glycemia and increases muscle GLUT 4 content in diabetic rats. Metabolism 46(7), 763-768 (1997) Jacob S; The antioxidant alpha-lipoic acid enhances insulin-stimulated glucose metabolism in insulin-resistant rat skeletal muscle. Diabetes 45(8), 1024-1029 (1996) Ziegler D et al. (1997) Alpha-lipoic acid in the treatment of diabetic peripheral and cardiac autonomic neuropathy. Diabetes 46 (Suppl 2): S62-S66

29. - Carnitine - Opie LH. Role of carnitine in fatty acid metabolism of normal & ischemic myocardium Am. Heart J. 97:375-388, 1979 Pola P. et al. Carnitine in the therapy of dyslipidemic patients. Curr. Ther. Res. 27:208 - 216, 1980 Rebouche CJ and Engel AG. Carnitine metabolism & Deficiency Syndromes. Mayo Clinic Proceedings. 58:533 - 540, 1983 Rossi CS & Siliprandi N. Effect of carnitine on serum HDL-cholesterol: report of cases. John Hopkins Medical Journal. 150:51-54, 1982 Sachan DS et al. Ameliorating effect of carnitine & its precursors on alcohol-induced fatty liver. Am. J. Clin. Nutr. 39:738-744, 1984

30. - Selenium Margaret Rayman, "Dietary Selenium; time to act", British Medical Journal, Vol. 314, 387, Feb 1997

31. - Zinc - Solomon, S.J. et al, Effect of low zinc intake on carbohydrate & fat metabolism in men. Federal Proc. 42 (1983), p.391. Tauri, S. Studies of zinc metabolism: Effect of the diabetic state on zinc metabolism: A clinical aspect. Endocrinology Japan 10 (1963), pp. 9-15 Faure P. et al. Zinc prevents the structural and functional properties of free radical treated-insulin. Biochimica et Biophysica Acta. 1994;1209:260-264

32. Madar Z, et al. Eur J Clin Nutr 1998;42:51-4

33. Diabetes Care 30:101-106, 2007

34. Am J Clin Nutr 2006 Jul;84(1):95-135

35. Kaprio J, Tuomilehto J, Koskenvuo M, et al. Concordance for Type 1 (insulin-dependant) and Type 2 (non-insulin dependant) Diabetes mellitus in a population-based cohort of twins in Finland. Diabetologia. 1992;35:1060-1067

36. Redondo MJ, Yu L, Hawa M, et al. Heterogeneity of Type 1 Diabetes: analysis of monozygotic twins in Great Britain and the United States. Diabetologia. 2001;44:354-362

37. Coeliac disease triples risk of Diabetes. Diabetes Care November, 2006

38. Hypponen E, Laara E, Reunanen A, Jarvelin MR, Virtanen SM. Intake of vitamin D and risk of type 1 Diabetes: a birth-cohort study. Lancet 2001;358:1500-1503

Index

Actos 59
acanthosis nigricans 33
albumin 41, 45, 50
alcohol 78, 112
Alzheimer's disease 55-56
antioxidants 29, 54, 80, 99-101
artificial sweeteners 76-77
atherosclerosis 47, 50-51, 71
Avandia 59
bitter melon 95
blood pressure 17, 24, 34, 40, 44, 47-48, 68, 84, 96, 98
body mass index 21
carbohydrate 14, 17, 26-28, 36, 60, 72-76, 82, 84
cardiovascular disease 40, 45, 85, 102
cataract 42, 48, 103
cherries 80
cholesterol 16, 24, 40-41, 45, 47, 59-60, 69, 70-71, 102
chromium 28, 96-97
cinnamon 95
coffee 80, 111
C-peptide 39
C-reactive protein 40, 55
creatinine 41-42, 45
depression 55-56, 92, 93
erectile dysfunction 32, 34, 51-52, 105
exercise 26, 35, 78-79, 86-89, 91
eye 28, 42, 45, 48-50, 102
fat 16-17, 21-23, 66-70, 79, 83, 85
fenugreek 95-96
fiber 27, 72, 80

food intolerance 156
fructosamine 39
garlic 96, 102, 104
genetic 19, 29-30, 155
gestational Diabetes 18, 30, 34, 38
ginseng 96
glaucoma 42, 48, 50, 102-103
glomerulus 50
glucagon 14-15
glucose - blood test for 35, 38
      challenge test 38
      tolerance test 36
gluten 156
glycemic index 73-75
glycemic load 73-74
glycosylated end products 29, 54, 80
glycosylated hemoglobin 38
glycosylation 49, 54, 80
grains 27, 72-73, 115
Gymnema sylvestre 94
HbA1c - see glycosylated hemoglobin
heart disease - see cardiovascular disease
hunger 17, 31, 63, 117
Hyperglycemia 47
Hypoglycemia 8, 47, 59, 87, 119-120
immune system 18, 55, 86, 104, 155-156
infection 32, 36, 55, 104-105, 156
insulin 14-17, 23-25, 36, 39-40, 46, 58, 64, 94-95, 155
insulin resistance 23-24, 27, 39
iron 97, 99
ketoacidosis 43, 47
ketone 42
kidney 41-42, 45, 50, 65, 76, 84, 103

lipoic acid 97-98, 103
liver 16-17, 59-60
magnesium 29, 80, 90, 93, 98
metformin 59, 79
nephropathy 41, 50, 65-66, 103
nerve damage - see neuropathy
neuropathy 53, 56, 98, 103
nitrates 99, 157
nuts 67, 72, 79, 100, 109, 117
obesity 22-24, 30
omega 3 fatty acids 28, 68, 157
oral Diabetes medication 58
pancreas 14-15, 38, 155
protein 29, 49, 62-66, 84-85, 106
retinopathy 49, 103
sexual dysfunction 51-53
skin tags.. 32
sleep 52, 88-90
stress 36, 90-91
stroke 48
sugar .14, 23, 27, 29, 35-36, 38, 43, 54, 70-75, 83-84, 115, 119
sulfonylureas 58-59, 61
Syndrome X 24-26, 32, 39, 78
testosterone 52, 105
thrush 32, 53
trans fatty acids 28, 69, 71-72
triglycerides 17, 24, 40, 45, 59-60, 71
twin 30, 155
viral infections 156
vitamin B12 59
vitamin D 93, 156-157
waist to hip ratio 21-23

Infertility:
the hidden causes

In this well researched book, Dr Sandra Cabot and naturopath Margaret Jasinska explore the many hidden causes of infertility which are often easily overcome.

One in six couples experience infertility. They are often left confused, hopeless and with no definitive answers as to what can be done to improve their chance of conceiving. Infertility is not a disease; rather it is a symptom of an underlying health problem.

By improving the health of both prospective parents, not only will this dramatically increase the chance of achieving a healthy pregnancy; it will also increase the likelihood of having a healthy baby.

In this book Dr Sandra Cabot and naturopath Margaret Jasinska help you to overcome problems that compromise fertility, such as:

- Endometriosis
- Balance your hormones naturally
- Overcome polycystic ovarian syndrome
- Overcome immune system disorders
- Reduce exposure to environmental chemicals
- Overcome hidden infections
- Vitamin and/or mineral deficiencies
- Understand tests you must have when trying to conceive

- Identify and overcome factors that lead to male infertility
- Increase sperm counts and improve the quality of sperm
- Improve your chance of success with IVF
- Maintain a healthy pregnancy
- Reduce the risk of miscarriage
- Give your baby the best possible start in life

This is what you will find at:

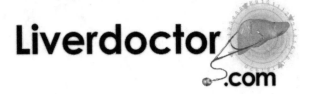

Holistic medical information

Well researched and up-to-date information to help you in your daily life
Informative on-line information to assist you look after your health and weight

Free liver check up test

Take this liver check up and receive private & confidential feedback on
the state of your liver and general health - www.liverdoctor.com/liver-check

Health supplements

Including Doctor Cabot's Livatone Plus capsules to support optimal liver function

On-line shopping

Sandra Cabot MD has a excellent range of health products and publications

On-line help from Dr Cabot's Team

Confidential and expert help from Dr Cabot's highly trained nutritionists and
naturopaths. Simply email us at ehelp@liverdoctor.com

Free LIVERISH newsletter

Register on-line for the free LIVERISH nesletter at www.liverdoctor.com/newslet

Love you liver and live longer

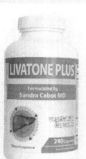

I am so glad I have been able to assist thousands of people to regain their health and vitality.

Sandra Cabot

Dr Sandra Cabot MBBS DRCOG

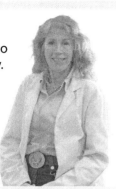

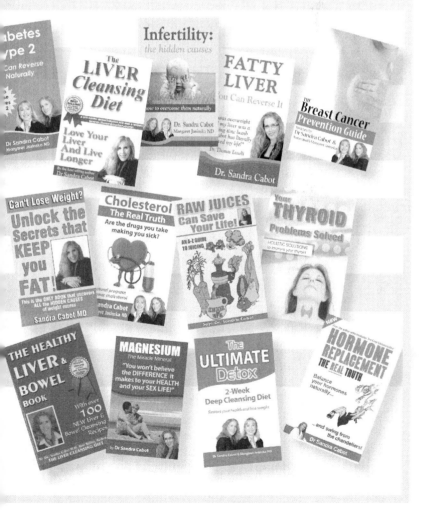

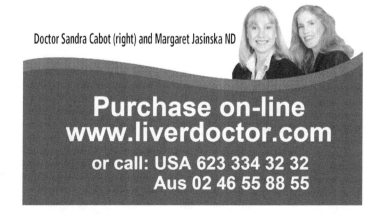